Innovations in Nursing Practice

Edited by

Kevin Kendrick

Senior Lecturer Philosophy and Health Care Ethics,
Liverpool John Moores University, Liverpool

Pauline Weir

Clinical Practice Development Nurse,
Royal Liverpool University Hospital, Liverpool

and

Elaine Rosser

Clinical Practice Development Support Nurse,
Royal Liverpool University Hospital, Liverpool

Edward Arnold
A member of the Hodder Headline Group
LONDON NEW YORK SYDNEY AUCKLAND

First published in Great Britain 1995 by
Edward Arnold, a division of Hodder Headline PLC,
338 Euston Road, London NW1 3BH

Whilst the advice and information in this book is believed to be true and
accurate at the date of going to press, neither the author[s] nor the publisher
can accept any legal responsibility or liability for any errors or omissions
that may be made.

British Library Cataloguing in Publication Data
A catalogue record for this book is available from the British Library

Library of Congress Cataloguing-in-Publication Data
A catalog record for this book is available from the Library of Congress

ISBN 0 340 60765 3

1 2 3 4 5 95 96 97 98 99

Typeset in 10 on 12pt Times by
Phoenix Photosetting, Lordswood, Chatham, Kent
Printed and bound in Great Britain by
J.W. Arrowsmith, Bristol

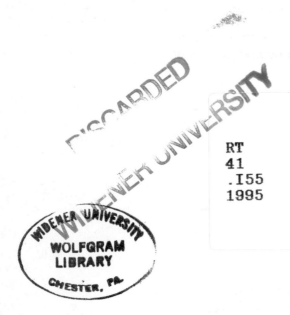

Contents

iv   *Contents*

List of Contributors

James William Brash RGN, Staff Nurse, Hope Hospital, Salford

Christina Hutcheson Dean RGN, RCNT, Dip Nurs (Lon), Ward Sister, Leighton Hospital, Crewe, Cheshire

Carmel Hale RGN, DPSN, BA(Hons), Clinical Nurse Specialist Innovative Practice, Fazakerley Hospital, Liverpool

Maureen Anne Hampson RGN, EN(G), DASE, DMS, Clinical Services Manager, Department of Medicine for the Elderly, Fazakerely Hospital, Liverpool

Patricia Ann Ingham BSc(Hons), RGN, Executive Director, Nursing, Human Resources and Quality, Tameside General Hospital, Ashton-under-Lyne

Terry Keen BA(Hons), DPSN, RMN, RGN, EN(G), Clinical Ward Manager, Clatterbridge Hospital, Bebington, Wirral

Kevin Kendrick MSc, BA(Hons), Dip Soc Admin, Cert Ethics & Theol, Cert Ed, FETC, RGN, EN(G), Ophthal Cert, Senior Lecturer in Philosophy and Health Care Ethics, Liverpool John Moores University, Liverpool

Nicola Catherine Leather BSC(Hons), Cert Ed, RNT, RSCN, RGN. Senior Lecturer in Psychology and Nursing, Liverpool John Moores University, Liverpool

Christine McKenna Auxiliary Nurse, Royal Liverpool University Hospital, Liverpool

Susan Thomas RGN, SCM, Clinical Practice Development Nurse, Royal Liverpool University Hospital, Liverpool

Stella Mary O'Gorman DPSN, RGN, RMN, Senior Commissioning Nurse, Broadgreen Hospital, Liverpool

Janet Lynne Richards RGN, DPSN, Ward Sister, Clatterbridge Hospital, Bebington, Wirral

Eileen Richardson RN, RM, ADM, Head of Midwifery, General Manager Obstetrics & Gynaecology, Fazakerley Hospital, Liverpool

Elaine Rosser RGN, RSCN, DPSN, BA(Hons), Clinical Practice Development Support Nurse, Royal Liverpool University Hospital, Liverpool

Thomas Shea MSc, DipHE, RGN, DNCert, Cert Public Admin, Macmillan Nurse Specialist, Broadgreen Hospital, Liverpool

Pauline Stitt RGN, RCNT, D/N(Lon), Cert Ed, RNT, BSc(Hons) Nursing, MBA (Health Executive), Principal Lecturer/Nursing Practice Development Manager, Liverpool John Moores University, Liverpool

Pauline Weir BA(Hons), RGN, DPSN, Clinical Practice Development Nurse, Royal Liverpool University Hospital, Liverpool

Foreword

This book is a fruitful product of a clear and sustained investment in nursing practice development by the nurses within the north west of England. The analysis of the clinical practice development nurse's role itself is excellent and an important contribution. The book flows with creative ideas, practical advice, hard won experience, honest reflection and sound analysis.

Each innovation is placed in its context. There is a meld of theoretical and personal experience and wonderfully telling case studies. Most of all you get the sense that these nurses really know from their experience of what they are writing; that they are deeply committed to providing a good service for patients and to the development and support of colleagues. The writing rings true as in the author who records that 'the rewards come from watching the development and true potential of others emerge . . . rather than from being Miss Fix It'; and the humour of the observation that 'reorganization of a busy Out Patient Clinic is rather like trying to service a car when it is being driven at 70 mph down the motorway'.

It is particularly encouraging to see these innovations flourishing and being supported in the new culture of the NHS and the book addresses how this is achieved.

This book is really worth reading and conveys the growth and energy of its authors; they are to be congratulated. I recommend it to you.

Susan Pembrey OBE RGN FRCN PhD
District Clinical Practice Development Nurse,
Oxfordshire Health Authority, 1978–1994

Section I

Section 1

Developing 'New' Nursing Roles

The emergence of 'new' nursing roles sets the scene for the innovations described within this book. As nurses are empowered to function in a positive and innovative way, development and expansion of their remit occurs. This yields practitioners who are willing to challenge the dogma and barriers to patient-centred care. Ultimately, their vision is to change and develop practice as a means of achieving excellence and meeting client needs.

In the first chapter, Weir focuses upon a personal insight regarding the clinical practice development role. Until recently, there has been a lack of literature relating to practice development within nursing and attempts to remedy this are identified. An overview of nursing roles which have been embedded within clinical practice creates the setting from which this new role flourishes. A key remit surrounding the role is the influence upon change through the areas of facilitation, autonomy, empowerment, reflection and support. By addressing how the post seeks to operate in the organization, the reader is provided with practical applications in which the role can be interpreted.

Building upon this, a chapter by Ingham and Thomas follows a similar thread within the growing area of practice development. However, this chapter brings with it a manager's perspective in addition to the practitioner's. It places particular emphasis upon identification of the directorate needs and how the role has endeavoured to meet these. A major aspect of this chapter surrounds the rationale regarding the expansion of the nurse specialist/advanced practitioner into a practice development role.

A lecturer/practitioner role is explored by Stitt, demonstrating the value of educationalists and practitioners working as partners within the nursing profession. Central to this, the author has been instrumental in developing the joint appointment from an educational perspective. An historical overview highlights the urgency of developing the role in the current academic and health service climate. Opportunities and difficulties emerging from the role are discussed by adopting a practical application, whilst an ongoing formative evaluation seeks to facilitate the role's development.

Finally, the emerging rheumatology nurse practitioner is examined in great detail by O'Gorman, giving insight into its application in other parts of the world. A description of how the author actively researched the role of a nurse within rheumatology is highlighted, with a brief account of hospitals and units visited. A resumé and critique of the findings during these visits culminates in the reasons for developing the role within the author's practice setting. Future developments are discussed and recommendations regarding changes in treatment; links with the community and staff education are put forward.

The Editors
1994

1 Clinical practice development role: a personal reflection

Pauline Weir

A leader is best when people barely know that he exists
Not so good when people obey and acclaim him
Worst when they despise him
Fail to honour people
They fail to honour you
But of a good leader who talks little when his work is done his aim fulfilled they will
  all say we did this ourselves

(John Adair, 1990)

The National Health Service (NHS) has witnessed many changes since its inception in 1948. However, the recent political philosophy of the 1980s has influenced new managerial themes and approaches. Emerging from this has been an agenda for devolved accountability and reduced hierarchy within hospital and community settings (Griffiths Report, 1983). The introduction of general management, the internal market and trust status has challenged nursing as the profession moves into the next century (*Strategy for Nursing*, 1989; *Vision for the Future*, 1993).

The ultimate vision for developing nursing practice should emerge from patient/client choice (*The Patients' Charter*, 1991 and *Vision for the Future*, 1993). The new nursing roles which are being created and developed must meet changing health care needs and with it, a needs-led service (*The Health of the Nation*, 1992). Finite resources and infinite demand will continue to dominate health care into the next century. For this reason, it is only in developing and changing health care practice and new nursing roles that the best use can be made of available resources. The 1990s brought with it an economic recession and put value for money on everyone's agenda, nursing being no exception.

The new culture within the NHS challenges nurses to develop their leadership skills and ensure nursing remains at the forefront of health care delivery. This chapter will concentrate on this 'new' culture and address a number of key issues relating to nursing and clinical leadership:

- Firstly, both the professional and national influences which have developed the clinical career structure in nursing over recent years will be examined.
- Secondly, the author will discuss the advancement of the clinical practice development role and its influence upon change through the areas of facilitation, autonomy, empowerment, reflection and support. All of these themes will be illustrated and examined through the application of case studies.

- Finally, the author will reflect upon the positive and negative aspects of the role and its function in relation to the wider organisation.

Clinical nurse specialist role

To date, mainly due to lack of role clarity and recognition, little has been written specifically around practice development roles. However, much has been cited over the years regarding other clinical roles, for example, the clinical nurse specialist (Castledine, 1991) and the consultant roles (Wright, 1990) and, more recently, advanced practitioner and clinical leader roles (PREPP, 1990). The development and scope of these roles will be reviewed as a means of explaining the emergence of the practice development role.

Much of the literature refers to the clinical nurse specialist as being the earliest type of clinical career advancement (Castledine, 1991). Historically, the role was established to improve nursing practice and so improve patient care. However, a combined initiative between medicine and nursing in 1970 established the Joint Board For Clinical Nursing Studies (JBCNS) which provided a systematic framework for post basic clinical courses for nurses. Pembrey (1989) saw the JBCNS as creating 'some development of specialist knowledge; specialist nursing and the possibility of some embryonic clinical careers'. This gave focus and direction to a developing theme.

Castledine (1982a) refers to the 1970s, within the Royal Marsden Hospital, in which many nurses were working in the field of stoma care, infection control and intravenous infusion under the term nurse specialist. Many hospitals followed the same route, giving nurses the opportunity to expand their role as they increasingly began to do the work previously undertaken by medical practitioners. The Royal College of Nursing pioneered the concept of the clinical nurse specialist role in the UK (Briggs, 1972). It first made such recommendations to the Committee on Nursing in 1971, following the earlier establishment of the post in both the USA and Canada.

The study by Castledine looked at the role of the nurse specialists and compared their development in the UK and other countries, mainly the USA. He identified two types of specialist nurse, 'those who perform a particular technical skill very well, and those who have developed a broader and more in-depth knowledge of clinical nursing practice'. He also highlighted three major factors which had precipitated their development:

- the increased demand for better services;
- the increased clinical content of nursing;
- the large number of nurses doing work previously undertaken by doctors (Castledine, 1982b in Markham, 1988).

Nevertheless, he discovered a lack of agreement about their exact function.

With the increasing interest in nurse specialist posts, the RCN set up a working party to look at the development of the 'Specialities in Nursing' (RCN, 1988). The group clarified the distinction between a nursing speciality and a nurse specialist. A nursing speciality means a field or component of nursing in which nurses may find themselves, whilst the nurse specialist refers to an expert in a particular aspect of nursing care (prepared beyond the level of registration).

Many authors have continued to examine the nurse specialist role and clarify their remit on both sides of the Atlantic (Markham, 1988: Morath, 1988: Storr, 1988: Brieger et al., 1989: Casey, 1990: Wright, 1991; Hotter, 1992). They all agree on the practice, educational, consultancy, research, management and administrative content of the clinical nurse specialist role. The RCN's report in 1988 concluded 'if the nursing profession is to reach its ultimate goal of providing relevant nursing care to meet individual patient's needs, then ultimately the role of the nurse specialist is central to its achievement'.

In 1988, Markham described two essential components within the clinical practice aspect of the nurse specialist role. Firstly, she described a direct care category consisting of assessing, planning, delivering and evaluating care. The nurse specialist acts as a role model, demonstrating expert knowledge and skills at an advanced level. Secondly, she highlighted an indirect category which encompasses the influencing, teaching, advice giving aspects of the role (Markham, 1988). This category also includes the setting of clinical standards and policies; and can be compared to the role of case manager (King's Fund, 1993).

Consultant role

Meanwhile, the 1980s saw the emergence of the term consultant nurse being used with increasing popularity in the nursing profession. Both Pearson (1983) and Wright (1986) identified the post as a continuum of the nurse specialist role. They emphasise that these nurses are practitioners directly involved in clinical practice as skilled change agents. Wright draws upon the work of Caplan (1970), who identified four types of consultations as follows:

- Nurse-centred (advice giving).
- Patient-centred (role model).
- Programme-centred (planning courses).
- Administrative-centred (advice on nursing practice and policy).

The term consultant nurse is likely to appear alien to many, but may be a natural progression for certain practitioners as their professional advice and skills are sought after throughout an organization.

In the last 10 years there have been many national and professional influences which have recognized and supported advanced nursing practice. The Cumberledge Report (1986) followed much unrest and disillusionment among nurses working in the community and acknowledged the need to enhance and develop their specialist skills. *The Strategy for Nursing* (1989) and the *Vision for the Future* (1993) set key challenges for the profession. Both promoted the identification of nurse leaders within clinical practice and recognized their value in the organization. Recently, the term 'named nurse' has become widespread since the establishment of the Patients' Charter (1991). The charter gave governmental approval to what nurses have been claiming is essential for high quality, individualized care. The UKCC recommendations regarding Exercising Accountability (1989), Code of Professional Conduct (1992a) and the more recent Scope of Professional Practice (1992b) have created avenues in role expansion and development in new territories of nursing practice. Finally, the proposals for Post-Registration Education and Practice within the UKCC which began in 1990 (PREP) seek to promote the continuum of nursing practice. The aim is to achieve this through preceptorship and clinical supervision leading to advanced and consultant practice.

Advanced practitioner

More recently, the term 'advanced practitioner' has been adopted throughout nursing practice and literature. The PREP document makes a clear distinction between advanced practice and simply working in a speciality. It describes specialist nursing practice as:

> practice for which the nurse is required to possess additional knowledge and skill in order to exercise a higher level of clinical judgement and discretion in clinical care and to provide expert clinical leadership, teaching and support to others. (*The Future of Education and Practice*, UKCC, 1993).

However, those prepared for advanced practice will be:

> equipped to assume the responsibilities of clinical practice leadership to meet patient, client and organizational need. (*The Future of Education and Practice*, UKCC, 1993).

The educational framework for specialist practice will focus on 'clinical nursing practice and programme management outcomes'; meanwhile, advanced practice will focus on 'clinical practice development and clinical practice leadership'.

To this end, the beginning of 1994 witnessed government support for the development of the nurse practitioner role. According to Casey (1994) 'nurse practitioners are pushing back new boundaries . . . not taking over what already exists; in the main they provide for what has never existed and that which nurses do best'. Examples of practitioners in these roles vary from nurse-led outpatient clinics, accident and emergency assessment and even responsibility for admission and discharge referrals. Casey concludes by stating 'it is a new era of practice which is recognised as different and complementary to medicine'. In the future, nursing care may be requested in its own right and the development of 'nursing beds' which evolved within Burford, Oxford will become an available and widespread option (Pearson et al., 1988). The admission of patients into hospital, primarily for therapeutic nursing care, validates that the nursing contribution in health care delivery has finally arrived.

Clinical leadership

The late 1980s brought the term 'clinical leader' into the nursing sphere. The Department of Health and Social Security submitted a report in 1988, to the NHS Management Board, Nursing Division, recognizing clinical leaders and their influence in the development of other nurses (DHSS, 1988). With this in mind, the nurturing of nurse leadership skills needs recognition, as according to (Holmes, 1991) 'since leadership appears to depend on the ability to influence others, this suggests that it may be the qualities of a leader that are important rather than the process of leadership *per se*'.

The mention of leadership, in whatever arena, automatically refers to management in certain organizations. However, the two should not be confused with each other. Management is about controlling, guiding and making sure things are done. Conversely, leadership is about directing, facilitating and influencing others. We need both leadership and management in an organization, but the organization will not be successful if the leadership qualities are absent.

For nurses to become leaders in clinical practice there must be both evidence of and an opportunity to develop certain leadership characteristics. Bennis (1989) argues that the basis of leadership involves having a guiding vision, passion, integrity, trust, curiosity and daring attributes. Meanwhile, Covey (1990) goes on to describe continual learning, being service orientated, radiating positive energy and believing in people, as other key leadership characteristics. Any organization undergoing major change needs people with these qualities. Nursing practice has to change and develop to meet consumer demand, and therefore those with the leadership skills must develop and empower others to achieve the same. Nevertheless, management needs to exercise empowerment at all levels within the organization as a means of influencing practice. The introduction of the new NHS and its devolved hierarchy is an attempt to facilitate this empowerment and ultimately address change.

Clinical practice development role

One of the disadvantages in widening the gate to clinical career opportunities has been the emergence of unclear titles which have tended to overlap existing roles.

However, the term 'clinical practice development role' was first cited in 1978 within Oxford, following the creation of a District Clinical Practice Development Nurse post. Unit Clinical Practice Development Nurse posts were later established throughout the region during the 1980s. Pembrey (1991) says the remit of their role centred on being 'responsible for facilitating the advancement of professional nursing practice in a unit. This work was mainly achieved through facilitating and encouraging others, through self-growth, to develop clinical practice'.

Pembrey highlights that the role has changed since its inception and identifies three broad categories for its interpretation as follows:

- *Change agent role* – 'this role is concerned with facilitating the process of change, rather than the substance of change . . . involves development skills and has a professional rather than a managerial focus'.
- *Specialist or consultant role* – 'this role offers particular clinical, educational or other expertise . . . this expertise may be provided in the employing unit or to other units within the authority'.
- *Professional or clinical leader type role* – 'these are people who create the visions . . . who inspire people to develop . . . help people plan . . . take practical steps towards shared goals' (Pembrey, 1991).

The next part of the chapter will draw upon the work of Pembrey and examine how the post has been interpreted within the Royal Liverpool University Hospital.

Practice development role in Liverpool

The author was one of the first practitioners to adopt the post in mid-1991, amidst three major changes which were influencing the hospital:

- Firstly, the hospital had recently gained Trust status and a department for nursing practice development was established.
- Secondly, the School of Nursing, previously within the hospital, had moved into a higher education arena and left the unit with an absence of on-site educational input.
- Finally, the publication of the Department of Health's Strategy For Nursing envisaged greater role flexibility to satisfy consumer demands by highlighting 'new roles which should be developed for practitioners to meet changing health care needs, improve care provision and realise the potential of clinical practice' (*Strategy for Nursing*, 1989). This continued to be expounded in the Royal Liverpool University Hospital's *Strategy for Nursing* (1992–1993 and 1993–1994) and in the more recent *Vision for the Future* (1993).

The clinical practice development role was developed to ensure that the Trust fulfilled the nursing contribution within its corporate objectives. The role is essentially a dynamic post in the sense that it will evolve and change, depending upon the demands within the organization. The role links with clinical areas to help facilitate an environment in which both nurses and practice can grow and develop.

Defining roles and their remits is not simple. The term 'clinical practice' refers to patient contact and patient involvement. An important aspect of the role is clinical credibility and participating in direct patient care, although not necessarily carrying a patient caseload. The attributes of a facilitator, resource person, educator and change agent are needed.

The 'development' aspect of the post encompasses both nurses and practice. Growth and advancement of nursing widens the boundaries of professional practice. This, in turn, leads to the maturation of practitioners who have experienced empowerment and been allowed to take risks and challenges through developing nursing. Issues surrounding empowerment, facilitation, and autonomy which operate within the post will be addressed in more detail later.

From a subjective basis the role has a broad remit which covers four areas:

- Providing individual clinical areas with support and a resource in which practices can develop and change according to the needs of the ward or unit.
- Facilitating the implementation of change (both the management and the process) by working with and on behalf of directorate/clinical managers.
- Empowering both staff and patients/clients to deliver or receive a nursing service conducive to a healthy lifestyle.
- Promoting the professional development of nurses.

Finally, the role is a staff and not line position within the nursing team and therefore carries no managerial responsibility. The essence of the role focuses purely on developing both nurses and nursing practice.

Prerequisites for the role

The characteristics of a clinical practice development nurse is analagous with any organizational development person. Chisnell (1990) devised her own 'Idiosyncratic List of the Necessary Qualities of a Professional Development Person' and this can be summarized as follows.

Individuals will:

- Want to do a good job 'for its own sake' and be prepared to take risks. This can be likened to the practitioner who develops individualized care despite the extra financial resources and increases to skill mix.
- Be pragmatic thinkers, who have the necessary knowledge and expertise in their area of practice to function independently. Reference can be made to the clinician who acts upon research findings and implements change against opposition.
- Believe in the worth and value of people and never under estimate the potential of the human resource. Examples of this can be seen in the implementation of a primary nursing approach to care and the changes in role specification around care assistants and nursing auxiliaries.
- Accept constructive criticism and act positively on receiving it. Nurses need to feel safe when developing practices and know that change may not always improve care.
- Network within and outside their organization and will gain satisfaction from seeing others succeed. This concept is new to nursing and is a valuable tool for the continued growth in nursing leadership.

Thus, the qualities of a development person and a leader can be seen to overlap and intermingle. Nevertheless, these attributes need to be exposed to nurses as early as possible in their careers. In doing this, we will enable nurses to challenge outdated practices and meet patient or client needs.

In the next section of the chapter the author will discuss the application of the post through the areas of facilitation, autonomy, empowerment, reflection and support when addressing change. A case study approach will be used to give insight into the role.

Application of the clinical practice development role

The last part of this century has brought with it major changes and advances in technology, political reforms and fluctuations in human resources. The nursing profession cannot escape the influential consequences of the development and innovation in the 1990s. Change is central to clinical leadership and a key remit within the clinical practice development role.

The *Concise Oxford Dictionary* (1990) defines change as 'an act or an instance of becoming different. An alteration or modification in someone or something'. Wright (1990) describes the term change as 'an attempt to alter or replace existing knowledge, skills, attitudes, norms and styles of individuals and groups'. Meanwhile, a change agent may be an impetus for the change, the instigator or the facilitator for change.

Facilitating change is pivotal to the role of the clinical practice development nurse. The ability to create an environment in which to pioneer innovations and 'make things happen' unites these practitioners and identifies leaders. Facilitating change and developing practice are synonymous within nursing. The following case study demonstrates how change through facilitation can take place in the clinical area and ultimately develop practice.

Case study – facilitation

Four ward managers shared an interest in developing patient self-medication in their ward, except none of them knew about each other. All had spent a considerable amount of time reviewing the literature and visiting places where this practice was happening. Each of them felt as if they were going round in circles and achieving nothing constructive.

The clinical practice development nurse, through working in each of the clinical areas, became aware of these similar stages of development. Comments of 'I didn't know Sister . . . was interested in developing self-medication!' 'How far has ward . . . developed this practice?' and 'How much support is ward . . . getting from the medics?' were made. Support was available in the form of someone who could look at the situation objectively and prevent each of the ward managers from re-inventing the wheel (an important issue in practice development).

A facilitatory approach was adopted to deal with this aspect of change. The clinical practice development nurse liaised with each of the ward managers and a self-medication group was established. There was mutual agreement to develop one protocol to bring about the implementation. The change agent provided the education and the resources in which to construct the protocol. However, the change in practice was a re-educative process, as ultimately the ward managers put the development into practice and in turn became the real change agents.

Discussion

For change to become lasting and permanent, an alteration in peoples' beliefs and values is paramount. The case study describes the change agent or clinical practice development nurse as facilitating the change. The change agent liaises and works with the group and becomes aware of the decision-making process. However, the recognition of the need for change and ownership comes from the practitioners wanting the change. This type of change can be likened to the normative–re-educative strategy or 'bottom-up' approach described by Wright (1990). 'Information and directions may be provided by the change agent when asked for by the group. The change agent may delegate change and offer minimal input as an individual from within the group adopts the change agent role' (Bennis et al., 1976; Hersey and Blanchard, 1982, cited in Wright, 1990). The impact of this approach to change will depend on the need for change from the individuals concerned. The case study demonstrates how, through facilitation, nursing practice can change and grow.

In addition, change requires levels of empowerment and autonomy to be experienced. Both of these concepts are also key traits within clinical leadership. Empowerment, as defined by the *Concise Oxford Dictionary* means, 'to authorize, license, give power to and make able or enable'. Meanwhile autonomy can be defined as, 'self-government and independence' (*Concise Oxford Dictionary*, 1990). Pearson (1983) says, 'autonomy refers to the freedom to make decisions within limits of the competence of the individual'. With reference to nursing he states, 'autonomy is about the power to act independently when those functions which are uniquely nursing are demanded by the patient's needs'. Vaughan (1989) goes on to argue that, 'there is a fine line between the freedom to practise autonomously and total freedom of action, which could generate into anarchy if we are not careful'. In the words of Henry and Pashley (1990), 'full autonomy is an ideal notion and we can only approximate to it'. Therefore, it can be argued that true autonomy at clinical level can never exist, as nursing practice is governed by carefully developed protocols which attempt to cover every eventuality. This is a symptom not only of nursing, but any bureaucratic organization.

Nevertheless, managers need to empower practitioners at all levels within the organization to develop and change the service according to client demand. Empowering nurses leads to the freedom to act within the boundaries of competence and enable a degree of autonomy to exist. The next case study looks at how levels of empowerment and autonomy can exist when change is introduced through a power-coercive approach (Wright, 1990). It demonstrates how the clinical practice development nurse can empower and encourage autonomy within the profession despite the bureaucracy.

Case study – empowerment and autonomy

Difficulties exercising empowerment and autonomy can arise when management introduces change through national and professional directives.

This was a situation an organization experienced with regard to inaccuracies in patient/nursing records. As a result, the nursing documentation needed to be urgently addressed. The recent reports from the Department of Health and the UKCC had made the initial impetus for change essentially a top-down strategy to improve record keeping (NHSTD, 1993).

In order to deal with this problem, an action group consisting of practitioners, managers, researchers and educators was formed. The group was chaired by a clinical practice development nurse who steered the group and the planned change. Awareness sessions and a teaching programme were devised by the group for the organization. Eventually, the involvement of the clinical practice development nurse in all the directorates (one per directorate) helped design the new documentation and both facilitate and manage change. A new form of documentation was developed and had ownership at clinical level, but the impetus for change had evolved from management.

Discussion

The case study showed how levels of empowerment and autonomy can exist when change is introduced through a power or coercive approach. This type of strategy is mainly used if a sudden or instant change is required. 'The change agent may provide information, give orders, direct change and even define the who, what, where, when and how the change will be implemented' (Bennis et al., 1976; Hersey and Blanchard, 1982, in Wright, 1990). This approach is essentially a 'telling' or 'top–down' style of change which is often used in bureaucracies. Nevertheless, the skills of the clinical practice development nurses enabled the new style of record keeping to be designed at clinical level by practitioners who would be using it. The role seeks to empower nurses despite the constraints of the organization and professional bodies. The degree of autonomy can be seen when practitioners have the freedom to take risks and develop new methods of record keeping which is not imposed from the managers. Total empowerment and autonomy may never truly exist in any organization, but practitioners can seek to exercise these concepts to meet patient/client needs (Henry and Pashley, 1990).

A fourth key characteristic within clinical leadership surrounds the concept of reflection. Reflection 'is about examining and exploring all aspects of your practice and goes far beyond merely evaluating patient/client outcomes' (Distance Learning Centre, 1992). As Coutts-Jarman (1993) says, 'people think about what has happened to them in a certain way, ponder upon events and draw conclusions. Working with experience in this way and using it to develop oneself is an important part of learning'. The reflective process involves analysing why something happened while it is happening, what was used, what was the result and includes how people felt about the incident. The third case study looks at the reflective process with regard to the management of pain.

Case study – reflection

While delivering patient care in a busy clinical area, the author became aware that staff were dissatisfied with the prescribing of pain relief for terminally ill patients.

An opportunity arose to examine this issue with the staff at the weekly ward meetings. The problem was identified as the inadequate prescribing of analgesia by junior medical staff. It was noted that every time junior doctors commenced on the ward, the nursing staff had to re-educate the doctors as to the most appropriate and preferred regime. They also felt that patient involvement in assessing and evaluating pain relief was poor and in some cases did not exist.

The clinical practice development nurse needed to convince the staff that they could contribute to resolving the issue and it was not solely a medical problem. Nurses could improve the way analgesia was prescribed and increase the quality of care. The ward was provided with empirical evidence regarding the successful use of pain assessment and self-recording charts. It was hoped the staff would be motivated to set about changing practice and devise their own pain assessment tool.

After spending considerable time reviewing the pain charts which were used locally, the staff did create their own. The form was designed so that it could be completed by either patient or staff, depending on individual patient needs.

Eventually, the medical staff used these tools for pain assessment and evaluation in prescribing patient analgesia. The ward has yet to evaluate whether patient involvement actually reduces the administration of analgesia. On reflection, the nurses believe that this change in practice has had the desired effect.

Discussion

'The reflective process unquestionably demands both critical thinking and self-awareness on the part of all practitioners' (Distance Learning Centre, 1992). They go on to state 'it requires them to question and, where appropriate, modify their perceptions of specific problems and to conceive innovative ways of tackling them'. The case study shows the practitioners reflecting on current practice within the ward environment. The author selected the ward meetings to provide an informal arena in which to encourage reflective practice. According to Darbyshire (1993), 'reflecting needs time if the recollection, sharing and discussion of stories and clinical encounters are to be undertaken seriously ... As much time as is currently allowed for managerial or administrative meetings'.

The third case study used reflection in changing nursing practice. The process of change involved a 'selling' or influencing approach for example, with empirical evidence. Here, 'the change agent provides the information and attempts to convince the group of the need for change' (Bennis et al., (1976) and Hersey and Blanchard, 1982, in Wright, 1990). According to Wright, this approach utilizes elements of both the 'bottom-up' and 'top-down' strategies. In the example, the reflective process changed practice through the development of a pain assess-ment/evaluation tool.

Growth of the post has mushroomed within Liverpool, with many directorates employing a clinical practice development nurse (*see* Chapter 2). These nurses have become identified as clinical leaders and form a clinical leaders' forum. The forum creates an avenue for peer support and the mutual sharing of ideas, devel-opments and innovations. Support is crucial if leaders are to survive in any orga-nization and the following case study describes how influential the support can be.

Case study – support

Certain practitioners wanted to operate single nurse drug administration in their unit as a means of continuing an individual approach to care. However, managers were reluctant to develop the practice, fearing the increase in drug errors. The issue was voiced within the clinical leaders' forum and soon became an agenda item. Once raised, other practitioners showed enthusiasm and a willingness to pursue the change. The clinical leaders displayed unified support and single nurse drug administration was explored by everyone. The findings were made available to management, who in turn, agreed to pilot the practice in a chosen area.

Discussion

The case study highlights the valued support and encouragement shown by clini-cal practice development nurses. Their existence within the organization creates an open pathway for clinical decision making and changing nursing practice. The case study describes an eclectic approach towards change, while the support is highlighted as the main driving force. The case study mirrors the themes dis-cussed by Wright (1990) for example:

- The practitioners who originally pursued single nurse drug administration were trying to 'sell' their ideas based on research findings (empirical approach).
- The clinical leaders as a group operated within a re-educative style (norma-tive–re-educative or 'bottom-up' approach).
- Finally, the managers retained their power and controlled the group (power-coercive or 'top-down' approach).

The concept of change is complex. Therefore, change within the nursing pro-fession is complex also. When addressing change, it is vital that practitioners select a suitable strategy or framework to match the situation. The changing cul-ture of society and the NHS requires a new breed of practitioner with advanced skills and expert clinical knowledge. This new breed of practitioner can be likened to a change agent or visionary and can be exemplified in the clinical practice devel-opment role. The remaining part of the chapter will focus upon the benefits and barriers to the role and discuss its relationship within the organization.

Benefits of the role

The clinical practice development post displays many positive assets. Firstly, the role can create both opportunity and freedom to take 'risks' and develop nursing within a safe environment. Developments which are untried and untested may not always show improvement or benefit in patient/client care. With this in mind, nurses need to work in environments which create opportunities to explore new boundaries in confidence. If this is to be achieved they in turn, must not be afraid of saying 'It didn't work' or 'I was wrong'. A healthy workplace will value its staff by empowering and supporting them as new territories are investigated. In essence, the post can be seen as a step towards facilitating this environment.

Secondly, when exploring new practices, nurses should have the opportunity to visit other like-minded people and network both formally and informally. This can involve other organizations as well as one's own workplace. For this to happen, time and resources are necessary. It may not be possible for a ward manager or staff nurse to justify 'visits', when the clinical area is dependent on them for 'hands-on' care. Having access to a practitioner with the resources and opportunities to network provides an objective bystander with a panoramic view and thus prevents re-inventing the wheel.

Thirdly, the role provides an avenue to address problematic and thorny issues in nursing at the grass-roots. Nurses have complained and will continue to complain about the structure and function of nursing practice. The role and forum provide a channel of communication which can have direct impact on patient/client care.

Finally, it is envisaged the post will change as nursing and the culture of the NHS changes to meet consumer demands. At present, it is creating a clinical career pathway for nurses who want to stay near to patient contact.

Barriers to the role

From a subjective basis, the post is linked to clinical areas with no specific patient caseload or management responsibility. To some, developing and changing practice may create difficulties when not directly clinically attached to a ward or unit. To others, this allows the change agent to practice in a more flexible role.

Nevertheless, the role may appear both solitary and isolated at times, despite the peer support within the clinical leaders' forum. It can be likened to experiences of a single ward manager who has replaced the former sister/charge nurse role. The inability to share thoughts and feelings with close colleagues in a similar role is an omission which the clinical leaders' forum seeks to remedy.

Another disadvantage to the role may be the absence of role models in this area of practice. Current professional nursing journals are now repeatedly advertizing for practice development, nursing development, professional development and clinical leader type posts. The profession is recognizing that if nursing is to remain at the forefront of health care delivery, new roles, with adequate funding, need to be established.

In 1991, the first clinical practice development posts were sited in the Clinical Practice Development Team, later known as the Development and Training Department of Royal Liverpool University Hospital. Much of the work, from a subjective basis, has been in collaboration with the directorate of general medicine while working in this department. By linking with a clinical unit, it has been possible to remain a credible practitioner by participating in patient care within the ward team. The advantage of working with practitioners without a management capacity has been the ability to observe nursing practice and help identify needs or challenges objectively – 'from the outside looking in'. This in turn, can bring additional resources to an area.

Clinical leaders' forum

The clinical leaders' group formed following the adoption of the clinical practice development role and is viewed as the nursing voice within the organization. The forum describes itself as '. . . existing as a group in order to communicate a defined clinical element to the overall strategy for nursing within the Trust, so that nursing and nurses will provide expert patient-centred practice ...' (Clinical Leaders, 1993). They see the clinical leader/clinical practice development nurse as functioning in the following ways within the group:

• to be prepared to take a lead and be seen as a representative of their unit/directorate;
• to strive to promote constructive working relationships within and outside their unit/directorate;
• to be prepared to learn from others within the group;
• to identify, evaluate and promote research based practice;
• to share information within the group;
• to develop and support one another; and finally,
• to act as positive agents for change.

(Clinical Leaders, 1993)

Currently, the identified clinical leader may or may not carry the title 'clinical practice development nurse'; nevertheless, they are the designated practitioner who has a remit for developing nursing practice. The continued growth and advancement of the forum continues to empower the role and give nurses authority and responsibility governing clinical practice issues. Examples of this empowerment are shown by the forum delivering guidelines on preceptorship, clinical supervision, record keeping and single nurse drug administration for the organization.

However, the formation of the clinical leaders' group has not developed without adversity. The newly created forum was exposed to feelings common to any recently established group. Similarities with the 'Tuckman's Model of Group Life' processes (Tuckman, 1965) were experienced and offered a tangible resource in which to steer the group through the difficult but necessary stages, for example:

- The Forming Stage (what shall we do or what will be our agenda).
- The Storming Stage (it can't be done, I won't do it or we will not be allowed to do that).
- The Norming Stage (we can do it by setting realistic targets).
- The Performing Stage (we are doing it by achieving deadlines and objectives).
- The Ending Stage (time for reflection during the clinical leaders' 'time-out' sessions.

'Time-out' days provide legitimate space to analyse and think about nursing practice and its contribution towards health care. The group's terms of reference and future agendas were born from these sessions and in turn, have created a cohesive and mature forum. Within the context of a time-out, a SWOT analysis (Strengths, Weaknesses, Opportunities and Threats) of the clinical leaders' group was performed and the following analysis draws upon some of the key issues which were identified.

Strengths

Main strengths were recognized as having the opportunity, freedom and power to change practice within one's own clinical area by liaising and contributing to the group's activity. The group considered the dynamic effect of clinical experts, who were both motivated and committed to develop nursing practice, would be invaluable to the organization.

Weaknesses

In certain clinical areas, practitioners may have other roles in addition to clinical leader, for example ward manager. Difficulties may arise regarding time for meetings, discussions and seminars. If many of the members cannot attend the regular forums, the group may lack cohesiveness and direction. However, clinical areas which employed a clinical practice development nurse in addition to ward teams found greater flexibility with allocation of time. Another possible weakness is that the person with the 'loudest voice syndrome' may receive the most attention. To remedy this, 'ground rules', terms of reference and a strategy need to be distributed, agreed and acted upon.

Opportunities

Broad opportunities were to develop and change nursing practice within the organization. The forum could be both a powerful and dynamic tool, but more importantly must remain productive in achieving patient/client needs. Changes to areas of practice which are common to all clinical units are recommended as positive ways forward, for example documentation, equipment, policies or procedures. Selecting issues which all members are concerned with will serve to unite and cohere the group.

Threats

Fear of imposed external agendas, limited resources and unrealistic goals may be overcome due to a group's commitment to work as a team. The group needs to be accepted as a valid body of practitioners whose expertise is recognized by others in the organization. This can be achieved with representatives updating and liaising with senior managers. From a subjective perspective, the scope of professional practice and with it, the expanded role of the nurse (UKCC, 1993), and the principles of case management are seen to be issues for these dynamic change agents to address. In the past, the rule of thumb would have been to appoint a 'person' to implement the 'expanded role' or case management in isolation from everything else.

From challenge to change

This chapter has highlighted the clinical roles which nurses have carved and developed over the last 25 years. As both society and the culture of the NHS changes, it is imperative that nursing continues to remain at the forefront of health care delivery. One of the ways to achieve this has to be through nursing roles which empower nurses to become leaders and positive change agents. Change is an eminent characteristic of our time and not to change is to stand still.

Practice development is an evolving and dynamic role. The themes surrounding facilitation, empowerment, autonomy, reflection and support are pivotal to the post and to clinical leadership. The case studies have demonstrated how these concepts can be applied in practice.

To summarize, nursing and nurses have and will continue to be managed within the NHS. However, the time has come for the profession to generate nurses to become leaders as well as managers. In the words of Hotter (1992) 'true empowerment thus creates leaders, rather than experts with management skills'. This theme is succinctly reflected in the words of Castledine who said, 'by reviewing the history and progress of specialization in nursing and the development of advanced practice, we can see that clinical nursing has finally arrived – the prospects for the future are good indeed' (Castledine, 1991).

References

Adair J (1990) *Not Bosses But Leaders*, 2nd edn. London: Kogan Page.
Bennis W (1989) *On Becoming a Leader*. Bonn: Addison-Wesley.
Bennis WG, Benne KD, Chin R, Corey KE (1976) *The Planning of Change*. London: Holt Rinehart and Winston.

Brieger G, Foster-Smith D, Muenchau T (1989) One approach to quantifying the clinical nurse specialist role. *Nursing Management*, Critical Care Edition, Nov. 1989, 80I–80S.

Briggs A (1972) *Report of the Committee on Nursing*. London: HMSO.

Caplan G (1970) *The Theory and Practice of Mental Health Consultation*. New York: Basic Books.

Casey N (1990) The specialist debate. *Nursing Standard*; **4** [31]: 18–19.

Casey N (1994) New practice boundaries. *Nursing Standard*; **8** [19]: 3.

Castledine G (1982a) *The Role and Function of Clinical Nurse Specialists in England and Wales*. University of Manchester: unpublished MSc Thesis.

Castledine G (1982b) In: Markham G (1988) Special cases. *Nursing Times*; **84** [26]: 29–30.

Castledine G (1991) The advanced nurse practitioner, part 1. *Nursing Standard*; **5** [43]: 34–36.

Chisnell C (1990) *Idiosyncratic List of Necessary Qualities for an Organisational Development Person*. The Wirral Hospitals, Unpublished.

Clinical Leaders (1993) *Clinical Leaders Bulletin*. Royal Liverpool University Hospital, issue No. 1, Dec. 1993, Unpublished.

Coutts-Jarman J (1993) Using reflection and experience in nurse education. *British Journal of Nursing*; **2** [1]: 77–80.

Covey SR (1990) *Principle-Centred Leadership*. London: Summit Books.

Cumberledge Report (1986) *Neighbourhood Nursing – A Focus For Care*. Report of the Community Nursing. London: HMSO.

Darbyshire P (1993) In the hall of mirrors. *Nursing Times*; **89** [49]: 26–29.

Distance Learning Centre (1992) *Reflective Practice*. The Distance Learning Centre, South Bank Polytechnic.

DHSS (1988) *The Way Ahead: Career Pathways for Nurses, Midwives and Health Visitors*. A Report to the NHS Management Board, DH Nursing Division, Career Development Project Group. London: HMSO.

Griffiths Report (1983) *NHS Management Inquiry*. London: DHSS.

Health of the Nation (1992) *Health of the Nation*. London: DOH HMSO.

Henry IC, Pashley G (1990) *Health and Health Studies For Diploma and Undergraduate Students Health Ethics*. Lancaster: Quay Publishing.

Hersey P, Blanchard K (1982) *Management of Organisation Behaviour*, 4th edn, Hemel Hempstead: Prentice-Hall.

Holmes S (1991) Clinical leadership: a role for the advanced practitioner. *Journal of Advances in Health & Nursing Care*; **1** [3]: 3–20

Hotter AN (1992) The clinical nurse specialist and empowerment: say goodbye to the fairy godmother. *Nursing Administration Quarterly*; **16** [3]: 11–15

King's Fund (1993) *Glossary of Terms in Managed Care/Case Management*. London: Nursing Development Unit, King's Fund.

Markham G (1988) Special cases. *Nursing Times*; **84** [26]: 29–30.

Morath JM (1988) The clinical nurse specialist: evaluation issues. *Nursing Management*; **19** [3]: 72–80.

NHSTD (1993) *Keeping The Record Straight. A Guide to Record Keeping for Nurses, Midwives and Health Visitors*. NHS Management Executive. London: HMSO.

Patients' Charter (1991) *Patients' Charter*. London: HMSO.

Pearson A (1983) *The Clinical Nursing Unit*. London: Heinemann.

Pearson A, Durand I, Punton S (1989) The feasibility and effectiveness of nursing beds. *Nursing Times*; **84** [9]: 48–50.

Pembrey S (1989) *The Development of Nursing Practice: A New Contribution*. The Inaugural Lecture, Institute of Nursing, Oxford.

Pembrey S (1991) *The Developing Role of the Clinical Practice Development Nurse*. Guidance Paper, Oxfordshire Health Authority.

PREP (1990) *The Report of Post-Registration Education and Practice Project*. London: UKCC.

RCN (1988) *Specialities in Nursing*. A Report of the Working Party Investigating the Development of Specialities within the Nursing Profession. London: RCN.

RLUHT (1992–3) *Strategy For Nursing 1992–3*. Royal Liverpool University Hospital NHS Trust, unpublished.

RLUHT (1993–4) *Strategy For Nursing 1993–4 'Windows of Opportunity – Moving Towards Collaboration'*. Royal Liverpool University Hospital NHS Trust, unpublished.

Storr G (1988) The clinical nurse specialist: from the outside looking. *Journal of Advanced Nursing*; **13**: 265–272.

Strategy For Nursing (1989) *Strategy for Nursing*. A Report of the Steering Committee. London: HMSO.

Tuckman B (1965) Development sequences in small groups. *Psychological Bulletin*; **63** [6]: 384–99.

UKCC (1989) *Exercising Accountability*. United Kingdom Central Council For Nursing, Midwifery & Health Visiting. Advisory Document, March 1989.

UKCC (1992a) *Code of Professional Conduct*. United Kingdom Central Council For Nursing, Midwifery & Health Visiting, June 1992.

UKCC (1992b) *Scope of Professional Practice*. United Kingdom Central Council For Nursing, Midwifery and Health Visiting, June 1992.

UKCC (1993) *The Future of Education and Practice*. UKCC, Unpublished Paper submitted to Ministers.

Vaughan B (1989) Autonomy & accountability. *Nursing Times*; **85** [3]: 54–55.

Vision For The Future (1993) *Vision for the future*, The Nursing, Midwifery and Health Visiting Contribution to Health and Health Care, DOH NHS Management Executive, April 1993.

Wright S (1986) *Building and Using a Model of Nursing*. London: Edward Arnold.

Wright S (1990) *Changing Nursing Practice*. London: Edward Arnold.

Wright S (1991) The nurse as a consultant. *Nursing Standard*; **5** [20]: 31–34.

2 The unit based clinical practice development role: A practitioner's and a manager's perspective

Susan Thomas and Ann Ingham

Why, sometimes I've done six impossible things before breakfast.
The Mad Hatter
Alice's Adventures in Wonderland
Lewis Carroll

How many nurses could identify with this statement? Probably all of them at some time or another. This is often brought about by an unstructured reaction to events, rather than the result of a planned, systematic process. Managing and leading nursing means facing a multitude of decisions every day: building teams, liaising with interdisciplinary staff, practising advanced nursing, acting as a role model and developing nursing within the ward. The needs of a clinical nursing team are very varied and stretch the skills of any nurse leader. Over the years the nursing profession has attempted to solve this problem by the introduction of new roles. This chapter aims to present a new role being developed within a Liverpool Hospital, the Unit Based Clinical Practice Development Nurse (CPDN).

The chief aims of this role is to develop nursing practice and provide leadership for nursing. This post has evolved from the role of the Clinical Nurse Specialist (CNS), which was the first attempt to create an advanced nursing role beyond the ward team. This CPDN role has attained its current form in response to the contemporary, social and political climate and professionalization of nursing. The authors will explore the themes underpinning the development of the CPDN and its application within a clinical unit.

Background

History

In order to understand the elements of the Clinical Practice Development Nurse role, it is necessary to explore how leadership roles have developed in nursing; why nurses have felt the need to change roles and what functions these roles performed. This review is confined to the UK and USA and does not reflect the changes which have taken place in other areas. Advanced clinical leadership roles in nursing began in the USA in the 1940s. Before this time advanced nursing, beyond the role of head nurse (equivalent to ward sister in the UK), was directed toward roles in nursing administration, teaching and supervision rather than clinical practice (Loudermilk, 1990). In the USA, the role of the clinical nurse specialist (CNS) was created with the purpose of improving the quality of nursing care. The evolution of this advanced clinical leadership role was influenced by the depletion of experienced nurses, particularly after the Second World War. This was coupled with an expansion in funds for postgraduate programmes, a broadening of knowledge relating to health, technical advance and the increasing complexity of health care. The emphasis in CNS practice was expert clinical competency. Hildegard Peplau implemented the first programme, in 1954, and empowered nurses to become advanced practitioners. Since then, the remit of advanced clinical skills has been expanded to encompass the roles of consultant, teacher and researcher. In the USA, the CNS was able to provide direct, sophisticated nursing care and to act as a role model and resource to others.

Two decades later, the case for the introduction of CNSs in the UK rested on the need for nurses whose prime commitment and responsibility was patient care, but who also provided clinical leadership. This was prompted by evidence given to the Briggs Committee on Nursing for the introduction of a 'clinical nurse specialist', initially called 'nurse consultant'. They suggested a clinical role without management or other duties. This clinical nurse specialist would work with nurses to assess and plan care and explore nursing problems. They would pass on knowledge and expertise and act as consultant. This would involve developing new patterns of care, investigating specific problems of nursing practice, making improvements and publishing results. From the examples given in their evidence it appears that this role was envisaged as spanning hospital and community, and being concerned with a specific patient group. It is also apparent that the expectations in terms of education, research and consultation were perhaps less than is evident in the American literature, being based at diploma level. In 1975, the RCN once again reviewed the issue of CNSs, prompted by the failure of the Briggs (1972) and Halsbury (1974) reforms to provide a career structure within the NHS which would allow the development of a purely clinical role. This review suggested that the role of nurse consultant was the absolute goal and that the role of CNS was an intermediate role between sister and consultant. It was envisaged that both these roles would have no line managerial responsibility (RCN, 1975).

General confusion continued to prevail during the 1970s concerning the preparation, functions, responsibilities and placement of the CNS in the bureaucratic structure (Hamric and Spross, 1983). This could be partly because nurses in the two countries were undergoing different political changes and aspiring to different goals relevant to the environments in which they found themselves, but developing roles using the same name. British nurses did not yet have government backing to expand their role to any degree. Even after the publication of the Cumberlege Report (1986) the government were only just realizing the potential of the nursing services (Clay, 1987). The USA, on the other hand, was developing expanded practitioner roles and focusing on better educated nurses.

By the 1980s there was agreement in the USA that the four major role functions of the CNS were expert practitioner, consultant, educator and researcher (Morath, 1988; Brieger et al., 1989). Recently, the emphasis seems to have changed away from being direct care giver, as the profession considered how to obtain maximum use of a person prepared at Masters level and began to appreciate the full scope of professional practice. The American Nurses Association (ANA, 1976) published a statement on nursing practice which included a description of the education, roles, functions and needs of the CNS. This formalized operational definition offered a positive step in differentiating the CNS's role from other expanded roles. By 1981, 81 programmes were available in the United States which offered clinical speciality preparation but the majority of these had appeared after 1972. In the United States and Canada, a Masters level programme is usually the required qualification for a clinical nurse specialist role.

The term Clinical Practice Development Nurse (CPDN) appears to have been used first in Oxfordshire in 1978 (Pembrey, 1991) for a role within the district health authority which was concerned with facilitating clinical teams to develop practice. During the 1980s the role became more common and unit based CPDNs were appointed. Pembrey (1991) states that the roles which the CPDN needs to perform to meet the current needs of nursing in Oxfordshire are: generic change agent; consultant with specialist skills; and professional leader. The CPDN role in Oxfordshire has never been a line management role and the focus has been mainly on educative activities in the broadest sense. This is quite different from the role mix described in the CNS's role history.

Ashurst et al. (1990) developed a role of Clinical Nurse Specialist Manager (CNSM), which has a high clinical profile while retaining a small management component. This is intended to help with the representation of the nursing team's bid for resources. The CNSM manages a sub-unit of two to four wards on a day-to-day basis, ensuring that staff receive adequate supervision, support and resources. The CNSM carries out individual performance review and participates in the development of in-house training programmes at ward level. This is another example of the evolution of a role to provide leadership for the development of nursing in the current post-grading, post-NHS reform climate in the UK.

As Hamric and Spross (1983) suggest, many of the early writings on the role of the CNS in the 1950s and 1960s were speculative, with general statements about definitions and qualifications, and there were few concrete role definitions described. Various names such as nurse clinician, clinical associate, liaison nurse and clinical supervisor were used. Lewis (1970) introduced her book on the clinical nurse specialist with the statement 'No one is yet quite sure of exactly who the CNS is, how she should be prepared, what are her functions and responsibility, where and how she fits into the institutional and agency structure'. During the 1980s the literature on the CNS had become more scientific and theory based. It had moved away from the need to describe role implementation from an individual's view point to more evaluative research of the role and more patient centred clinically orientated articles. Such developments reflect a growing awareness that it is not the role title which matters, but that the role mix fits the environment in which it is situated.

Roles

Hamric and Spross (1983) describe the CNS as 'an expert clinical practitioner who functions in a specialised area of nursing, who has expanded authority and autonomy, and who directs her efforts towards the improvement of patient care and practice'. She identifies direct care giving as a major function and also the ability to act as a change agent within the health care system. Mayo (1984) described the CNS as an expert practitioner because she or he has a broader knowledge, deeper insight and greater skills than those acquired in a basic nursing course. There is, therefore, the added expertise to analyse, explore and cope with nursing situations within and beyond a specific clinical field. Noll (1987) contends that the main task of the advanced role is problem solving and effecting planned change, but it is suggested that this perception has only recently begun to take root and many post holders value the hands on clinical aspect of the role. The role of change agent has now emerged as the key issue in advanced positions, and, it could be argued, is central to the development of the CPDN (Antrobus and Whitby, 1994). However, before exploring this issue, it is important to understand the range of aspects which have been ascribed to the emerging role of CNS, since it is from this that the vision of the CPDN has grown.

The literature (Cox, 1978; Hamric and Spross, 1983; Storr, 1988; Boyd et al., 1991) on this role supports Hamric's major categories and also describes sub-roles that include practitioner, educator, researcher and consultant. As the categories of sub-roles of the CNS role emerged, advanced clinical competence was no longer the only or even the main aspect of the role of the CNS. The role was defined differently in various locations which created ambiguity and individual specialists were left to define and develop their own position within institutions. An advanced practitioner must be involved in direct care giving through assessing, planning, delivering and evaluating care. By demonstrating their abilities and enhanced competence, they act as role models for the other members of staff. They also retain their professional credibility by being seen to do what they advocate. Care not directly involving patients includes being active in setting, developing and measuring standards of care, developing and improving nursing practice, being a resource, providing information and promoting communication, all of which helps to demonstrate an acceptance of change and an ability to influence its course positively.

Loudermilk (1990) suggests that there are several sources of role ambiguity within the CNS role. These are: inadequate socialization to the role; conflicting role expectations of managers and staff; inconsistent job descriptions; poorly defined job qualifications; multiple accountability; inconsistency in placement within the bureaucratic framework and unclear criteria for evaluation. Inadequate socialization to the role is caused by a shortage of role models and peer support due to the fact that only a small number of nurses are working in this kind of a role. Conflicting expectations of the role between the managers and the staff arise due to differing perceptions and this may cause confusion over direct lines of accountability. The problem with inconsistent job descriptions is the need to define the role and yet allow for dynamism and change to meet the organization's changing needs. These factors make evaluation of the role difficult but vital.

Since the 1950s when the role of the Clinical Nurse Specialist (CNS) first began in the USA, the CNS has been expected to perform research. Martin (1990) suggests that the CNS should be a professional practitioner who could advance nursing practice via scientific research, and produce clinical nursing research. This expectation is evident in Peplau's statement in 1965: 'Clinical specialisation is also a basis for clinical nursing research. As the numbers of clinical specialists increase the clinical nursing research will also increase'. Most advanced roles are expected to contribute towards clinical research, but this expectation is rarely fulfilled. First, there is a wide variation in the scope, quality, focus and intent of research education. Research is time consuming and takes time away from direct care giving. The need to ensure quality patient care, provide staff education, participate in policy, procedure, standard setting and keep abreast of latest developments may have a higher priority than research activities. Institutional and departmental readiness to support research can vary. There may be administrative support for efforts at improving overall quality of nursing care but not the same support for formal research. Staff may not understand the value of a research project or the amount of effort that is involved. In addition to this, the advanced practitioner may lack confidence to do research. Research is the weakest area in the development of advanced roles, but it is an essential element if the profession is to develop practice on a scientific basis.

Clinical careers

The 'Clinical Advancement' or 'Clinical Ladder' concept recognizes that nursing is practised at several levels of skill and competence and that clinical nurses should be rewarded according to their levels of expertise. In the USA Clinical Advancement Programs encourage and reward nurses who remain in the patient care delivery role and motivate both new and experienced nurses to move to higher levels of practice, by increasing their skills and knowledge. The fundamental purpose is to provide a mechanism for recognition of nurses who advance their levels of practice.

In the UK the Clinical Career Structure presented by the RCN (1980) offered a career ladder moving from basic training to Nurse Consultant including specialism in General Care and Special Care which eventually became the NHS Nursing Clinical Grading Structure (Fig. 2.1). This sought to establish a clinical structure which was separate from Education and Management but was not very successful since the grading definitions mainly concentrated on qualifications and managerial responsibility rather than advanced clinical practice roles.

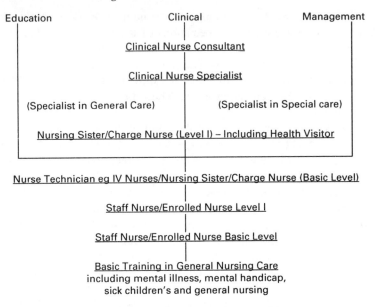

Fig. 2.1   Royal College of Nursing (1980)

NHS culture change facilitates development

In the UK several changes have taken place which have improved the climate for developing clinical nursing. Beginning in 1990 the advent of Hospital Trusts allowed organizations to gain autonomy over their practice, structures and reward systems (Ham, 1991). Services began to be defined through negotiation with purchasers and this in turn increased the flexibility to determine appropriate nursing teams and radical forms of care delivery. One of the key changes has been the development of the directorate structure which has brought about closer team working between different disciplines. Within directorates, some nurses now hold general management positions while others hold principally nurse management positions. Within the Royal Liverpool University Hospital Trust (RLUHT) directorates are managed by nurses in general management positions whilst each also has a clinical nurse leader. If this model is implemented elsewhere, it could lead to the split between Clinical Nursing Leadership and Management long desired by the RCN (1980). Several other factors also influence this situation. The publication of the *Strategy for Nursing* (DoH, 1989) and *Vision for the Future* (DoH, 1993) have highlighted key nursing development issues; the continuing work of the King's Fund in supporting and promoting Nursing Development Units and the Patients Charter requirement to practice 'named nursing'. All of these have been high profile national initiatives which have put nursing development issues on the main agenda at least for a time.

These changes taking place in the National Health Service have paved the way for new nursing structures and experimentation with roles and relationships (Salvage, 1990). Changes within the NHS have brought about the devolution of decision making responsibility and many roles have changed. Nursing, therefore needs to be flexible in making the most of local circumstances to enhance nursing care by using nurses appropriately. These are some of the reasons the CPDN role has developed in the RLUHT. The role has evolved from that of CNS and other advanced roles; it provides a new model for an advanced role which meets the needs of the current environment.

Clinical nursing leaders: a powerful body

The climate of change and devolved management creates the opportunity for clinicians to influence the shape of the service. Directorate Teams can determine what services they will offer and how they will organize those services. Prisk (1991) suggests that clinical nurse leaders should participate in formalized days to engage in professional development, peer review, evaluation of research and projects. Meanwhile in the USA 'Shared Governance' is giving clinical nurses power to determine organizational policy concerning nursing (Porter-O'Grady, 1987). The *Vision for the Future* (1993) requires clinical supervision and leadership to be established within nursing. This calls for each Clinical Nursing service to have a leader who is an expert nurse and probably an advanced practitioner. These nurses constitute a powerful force for change within their organization and outside it. Within the RLUHT, the opportunity has arisen to develop a clinical leaders' forum which gives CPDNs a network, a voice in organizational policy and provides the raw material for the development of clinical supervision.

The CPDN role

Creating a new role

In the summer of 1992, the role of CPDN was created in the Ear, Nose and Throat (ENT) Directorate of the RLUHT. Each ward had a ward manager whose role was evolving and becoming increasingly busy with managerial issues; this left little time to act as facilitator and role model. The CPDN role was created in addition to the ward manager roles, with no line management responsibility and a very flexible remit to facilitate nursing development. The post reports directly to the Directorate Manager, a nurse, who can see where nursing development will mesh with the organizational objectives and acts as support to the CPDN.

It could be suggested that leadership is very much like taking a space journey. Having been given the job and the equipment to do it, the final journey is filled with unforeseen mysteries. The destination is known but it is far away and is not a tangible reality. The basic skills have been learned but much of the learning process has to be undertaken *en route*. There is fear of the unknown and the worry that the demands will find the leader lacking. In the eyes of the crew, the leader must appear fair in decision making and able to meet challenges; even though the way may be long and hazardous and many unexpected surprises found on the journey; learning needs to be continuous and often there is no one to turn to for advice.

This describes very well the position of any leadership role in clinical nursing. The role is usually the only one of its type in the unit, and is prone to isolation. There is a need for the job holder to seek a flexible job description and objectives that allow for individual scope and development. The freedom to pursue personal endeavours and beliefs, and 'sort things out' needs to be tempered with an organized plan of action. Often role ambiguity becomes a real threat to undermining the efficiency and productivity of the CPDN. Effective management of time and freedom to set priorities are all essential to fulfil the role. The pressure that the role brings requires the job holder to cultivate and develop support systems outside the clinical area, and a well-developed networking system is worth promoting.

The expectations of others, both overt and covert, places unseen pressure on the person creating the new role. Within the ward environment, the emphasis is on maintaining clinical credibility and being seen to understand the problems faced at grass roots level. At managerial level there is the pressure to achieve visible changes.

Framework of responsibility

First, a suitable framework and broad outline of the responsibilities involved needs to be clarified. Placing a CPDN in a staff position instead of a line position makes the sphere of influence and responsibility dramatically different. The line manager has direct influence and contact with senior managers and the ability to influence practice. The CPDN in a staff position has less direct contact and influence with senior staff in managerial positions and requires an avenue to develop in which they can influence and change practice. As a group, CPDNs can become politically active and exert great influence in promoting improvements in care and influencing change.

The power to liaise with staff at executive level and voice the concerns and aspirations of junior staff requires a role holder who can act as advocate without the background of a managerial agenda. There is some disagreement in the literature regarding the placement of the advanced practitioner in the line or staff position (Morath, 1988; Storr, 1988). Staff placement enables the nurse to exert authority because of his or her expert knowledge and clinical competency. Freed of some organizational constraints, the advanced practitioner can concentrate on qualitative concerns relating to patient care. It should also be mentioned that collaboration with and support from managers are essential to function successfully in a staff position. The advanced practitioner may spend considerable time listening to frustrated or burned out staff members so a staff position supports a staff advocacy role more than a line position. However, a line position conveys positional and resource power which may be difficult to attain in a staff role.

The decision to create an advanced role within the nursing structure, free from line management responsibility, was made as a result of a previously introduced CNS post whose role became that of manager instead of clinician. The CNS role was created in 1988 and followed the RCN model, but the management component overwhelmed the clinical one. This was partly due to the previous experience of the post holders and the prevailing traditional management structure. The role was disbanded when the hospital obtained Trust status and Directorates created their own mini structures.

Components of the role

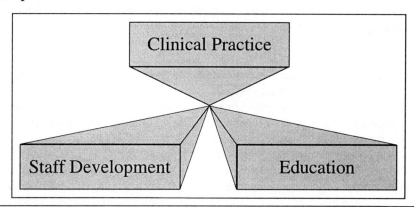

Clinical Practice
Communicate new role to staff on relevant wards
Maintain clinical practice
Act as patient/staff advocate
Attend ward/unit/directorate meetings
Challenge established practice
Publish work
Develop a culture that assists staff to work as a team
Promote research based practice
Act as a catalyst in the development of new ideas, etc.

Staff Development
Encourage cross fertilization by facilitating links with other areas
Involve staff in projects and action plans
Develop staff potential
Initiate support groups
Arrange orientation programmes

Education
Negotiate learning contracts
Arrange visiting speakers
Arrange teaching sessions
Update staff on developments in nursing
Assess educational needs
Give lectures, talks to conferences, groups
Act as proponent of good practice
Assist staff to develop teaching packages
Provide advice on nursing practice
Contribute to selection procedures
Assist in the appraisal process by helping staff to generate ideas, fulfil action plans and meet their objectives

Aims and processes

The role was first introduced to assist staff in providing and improving the quality and effectiveness of patient care. The three main aspects of the work involved clinical practice, education and staff development. It was envisaged that in enabling staff to provide expert clinical care, they themselves would need support, guidance, and assistance to develop them. Providing staff with a caring, learning environment was at the heart of the first year of the development. Developing the roles of staff within the unit was essential before anything else could be achieved. 'Time out' days were organized with the emphasis on team building, valuing each others' strengths and achievements and presentational skills. Later in the year, the focus moved to the provision of quality care and the result of patient satisfaction surveys.

The prime aim was to recognize the strengths and weaknesses of the directorate as a whole and this included all members of the multidisciplinary team. Different perceptions were held by staff within the directorate and this required recognition and discussion. Meetings were necessary on a regular basis to enable staff members to air their views in a structured way. Considerable time and effort were required in building relationships between staff so they felt safe in airing their views. The response from staff at having their views considered made up for the expense in time.

Empowerment

Following these consultations, further information was elicited concerning education, professional development, innovations and support needs. Armed with this information, realistic and achievable goals were formulated which would produce visible and rewarding outcomes. Thus commenced the first year's development plan. The main thrust was concerned with encouraging staff to become their own leaders and initiators. In creating a risk taking culture, it was necessary to encourage staff to make their own decisions. This was by far the most difficult philosophy to uphold. The senior staff had to hesitate from providing all the solutions and wait while staff discovered answers for themselves.

(Garratt, 1987) suggests that organizations with well established change orientated cultures actively enable staff to accommodate change more readily. The process of devolving management responsibility to the appropriate level gave staff a taste for authority and autonomy. At first it was met by fear, non-acceptance, and avoidance of change. Now, 3 years into Trust status, staff are becoming more aware of the hospital's changing culture and have seen the benefits of becoming actively involved in decision-making processes.

A central theme was the development of nurses' ability to practice innovatively and autonomously, and hence develop practice. The main means of achieving this was through facilitation rather than direct action. Offering this sort of leadership poses a unique challenge, as the leader strives to maintain a balance between setting goals and encouraging nurses to address their own agendas. There are always external pressures and deadlines to be addressed such as national and organizational strategies, but people do not learn autonomy and self motivation through being given detailed instruction in every move. Often it is necessary to allow mistakes, but some of those mistakes can result in penalties and this has to be weighed against the need to learn. One of the key issues is the personal qualities of the leader. A certain amount of drive and commitment is needed, tempered with patience and a genuine desire to see people develop professionally and personally. Creating a balance between impelling and facilitating has not been easy, especially as the balance must be dynamic to allow flexibility, but the balance is essential and has been managed carefully through collaboration between the CPDN and the Manager.

Staff development

Through creating an environment of facilitation and empowerment, staff are able to learn and develop at an accelerated rate. Practical experience combined with theoretical knowledge became the base of development. Development is infectious, and staff who previously have recoiled from undertaking a degree or conversion course have been encouraged by the success of others. Freedom to be able to arrange extra training and education of staff is an essential component of the CPDN's role. A training budget allows for the provision of outside courses and study days and it also allows for a degree of negotiation in the formation of training contracts between both parties.

Caring aspects

Caring for staff and facilitating in their development is fundamental to achieving support for change. The nurturing role of the CPDN can take many forms, from coaxing the development of a new idea or project, to supporting and giving confidence to members of staff in their pursuit of new skills. Enabling staff is a basic component of the role and underpins the basic philosophy of change management. The evolution of new ideas and developments is only the first stage. Making ideas a reality comes from providing a supportive environment and freedom to make changes. Devolving management structures are part of the enablement process. The CPDN is not there to provide solutions to the inevitable array of problems that surface throughout the day, but to provide the means by which staff can find their own solutions. It is very tempting to resort to providing a quick fix approach, or to be seen as knowledgeable about everything and able to provide all the answers. Appearing less than perfect when one has years more experience and a more senior position is more than a little daunting. The facilitation role counteracts the perceived failure to provide all the answers by encouraging staff to believe in themselves and by providing a supportive environment in which risk taking is actively encouraged and mistakes seen as something to be learned from. The role is very often isolated despite its appearance of being very people orientated. In providing support for a large number of staff, the role can become very fractional and one-sided. The job holder can often find the rewards are not clear cut and come in the form of watching the development and true potential of others emerge rather than the expressive thank-you's gained from being 'Miss or Mr Fix It'.

Preceptorship, as defined by the UKCC PREP (1990) project, provides ongoing and essential support for staff within organizations that are in a state of rapid change. It is important whilst involving staff in their own development to consider the aims of the organization and the CPDN is in the ideal role to marry together the personal aims of the staff and the needs of the organization. One of the ways this was achieved was by encouraging all staff to begin setting out their personal professional development profiles. This proved a valuable exercise in reflective practice and goal setting. With the aid of the CPDN each nurse was able to set out their personal aims in a structured way, interlinking these with those laid out in the directorate and hospital business plans.

Outcomes

Several important outcomes have already been identified from the work so far.

---

1   All staff have professional profiles.
2   The Directorate has made progress towards individualized, patient focused care.
3   The 'Ward Philosophy' has been expanded and developed into a multidisciplinary 'Unit Philosophy'.
4   Personal development plans which aim at individual goals have been developed.
5   There is an increased climate of development and desire to grow and learn and the uptake of post basic courses increased.
6   A budget for training staff has been identified.
7   There is low wastage of staff.
8   Time out days have taken place to determine strategic goals.
9   Information literature for patients has been improved and increased.
10 Staff have been updated in clinical developments and changes in nursing.
11 Relaxation and aromatherapy have been introduced.

Power and influence

The ultimate aim of the CPDN role is improving patient care. This can occur by empowering staff at grass roots level, but also by bringing about upward change. Clinical leaders at this level require an avenue to create change at executive levels. The formation of a pressure group of like-minded individuals will help to assist this process of upward influence. One of the ways in which this was introduced in the RLUHT was the formation of a Leader's Forum which arranged its own agenda and identified areas of practice which required restructuring or improvement. The group was made up of CPDNs who practise nursing and the natural clinical leaders of their clinical team. The group is still in its infancy but has already addressed such issues as preceptorship, patient documentation, drug administration and the expanded role of nurses. This group makes nursing policy for the organization in a form of shared governance, is very unbureaucratic and forms a network for influence internally and externally to the organization. Members of this group are also the main initiators of a regional clinical practice development network.

Evaluation of role implementation

Successes

One of the major satisfactions of this role has been contributing to the development of others and nurturing their development. It is very gratifying to see personal and professional growth in members of the nursing team. There is also a real sense that this growth is helping to improve patient care. Practice is changing and ideas are now being generated and explored. Promoting a climate of teaching and learning has been significant in bringing about this culture change. In addition to this the CPDN has been able to carry out the role in a way which maintains clinical expertise and builds up networks of contacts in managing and teaching roles which can be readily 'tapped' when expertise is needed.

Difficulties

One of the major problems with the role is organizing the time to enable the maximum benefit to be gained from it and achieve priorities. The role is diverse, has indistinct boundaries and involves supporting people in change; of these factors, time management is very challenging and stressful. For this reason, it is imperative to develop peer support systems outside the clinical area. This is difficult because of the small number of colleagues in this kind of role. The complexity of the role generates a considerable amount of guilt at not being able to do more. As previously described, the role addresses different expectations from a number of other people, both overt and covert, and it is often difficult to identify these expectations and prioritize. The structure of the role makes it difficult to achieve ongoing long term involvement with patients and this reduces the ability to practice and demonstrate management of patient care in the fullest sense.

Challenges

Alternating the use of time to reflect changing needs as the role develops is central to success. The role is dynamic and, looking back, constant reappraisal is required to cast off redundant activities and make room for new ones. This means that the role is never comfortable and can be very tiring, so it is important to allow time for reflection and to 'catch one's breath'. There is still a need to clarify collaborative relationships in order to maximize the contribution of the CPDN. One of the key objectives for 1994 was to assist staff to generate ideas and develop personal professional goals and action plans. This should result in a shift of emphasis in the CPDN role from supporting to empowering, from developing nurses to developing Nursing. This will help to cement individual responsibility for development, and match personal development with organizational goals. However, it is a complex process and requires the development of a proactive ethos which some individuals find very challenging.

Needs

As already discussed, there is a need to reassess activities regularly and this demands a flexible job description. So much change has taken place that clarifying goals and core activities has now become a priority. Likewise, objectives are agreed annually and need to reflect not only the aims of the directorate but also the needs and aims of the staff. There is also the need to renegotiate when new opportunities arise which require reprioritization of existing activities. The role now needs to move towards exerting more effort on developing practice and leave nurses to take responsibility for their own development within the framework of goals and action plans. Some of this can be achieved by informal networking throughout and beyond the hospital and also by sharing and joint working. The Clinical Leaders' Forum needs to be developed to become more vigorous and strong and the CPDN needs to join groups to work on projects and influence policy.

Enhancing autonomous practice and facilitating reflective practitioners is one of the key needs. One of the organizational goals is to move towards more collaborative care which embodies the ideals of 'case management' and 'patient focused care' systems currently employed in parts of the UK and USA. These ideals focus care around the patient and aim to ensure care is optimally sequenced and outcome based. If the gains in nursing care are to be maintained and developed, it is vital that the nursing team are able to practise with confidence and conviction and to articulate their goals and values to other members of the interdisciplinary team.

Managerial expectations – cost effectiveness

Obviously, there is a considerable cost involved in providing an experienced advanced practitioner in a senior grade for this role. There are considerable cost pressures within the organization and so the role must be seen as valuable within the wider organization. This generates a need for visible successes in terms of meeting external targets as already discussed. Demonstrated success in meeting the 'named nurse' target, reducing junior doctors' hours, identifying outcome measures, and developing a model of clinical supervision, gives the organisation tangible evidence of the value and effectiveness of the role. The CPDN must maintain a balance between these targets and the staff's current needs. The CPDN and the Manager form the interface between these two very different sets of priorities and perceptions of timescales. So far, a fairly good balance has been achieved through discussion and mutual adjustment of goals and plans, but the pressure does generate some dissonance and frustration.

Effects of culture change

There is a trend within nursing to resort to conformity and rigid frameworks, and in this, the ENT directorate is no exception. The new culture of encouraging personal initiative and responsibility came from the top of the organization and is filtering down. As demonstrated by Menzies (1960), there is a tendency in the old culture for upward delegation. However, in the current NHS, decision making responsibility is being rapidly devolved throughout the organization. Rapid change in organizations provokes anxiety and stress, and there is therefore a tendency for the team to regard the CPDN as a solution for problems, and an avenue for delegating problems upwards. They can also be seen as a stand in for staff who are sick and a knowledge bank who will provide the 'correct' solution.

The future

Is the role working?

As has been demonstrated, there have been several important and tangible outcomes of the role so far. There is also a less measurable, but detectable feel of increased energy and desire for progress within the team. Within the organization, the Clinical Leaders' Forum is seen as growing in confidence and influence. This provides a vehicle to incorporate the values of the 'New Nursing' (Salvage, 1990) into the development of Collaborative Care and Patient Focused Care across the organization and thus provides a voice for clinical nurses in strategy development. At the local level, the role is stressful and not always understood by the nursing team who are sometimes too close to the trees to be able to see the shape of the wood! However, several members of the team are beginning to take the initiative in creating change and developing practice. They are networking with other nurses and bringing fresh ideas and support to the team. This has engendered optimism and increased empowerment to improve care. In this respect the role has been effective in changing nurses and nursing.

Evaluation

Since the central goal of the role is to develop nursing practice, evaluation should seek to establish improvement in quality of care due to the impact of the CPDN role. Annual objectives form the basis for planning and evaluation. The objectives identify shared and sometimes conflicting priorities and become the focus for the dissonance between bottom up and top down expectations. However, even when consensus is reached, there remains the difficulty of expressing and measuring intangibles such as increased motivation, autonomy, patient participation and dignity. As identified in the literature, (Minter-Peglow et al., 1992), even where such changes could be audited, it is difficult to identify objectively the contribution made by the CPDN. Evaluation, so far, has therefore failed to identify concrete improvements in quality which are a direct result of the CPDN role, but this is partly because, as already identified, the role has been focused on the development of nurses in the initial stages not on Nursing Development.

Further, more rigorous evaluation of the role needs to take place. Minter-Peglow et al. (1992) suggest several methods of evaluation which may be of use. Structure evaluation data are objective and easy to evaluate and structural components can influence performance. However, structure evaluation has limited value because this approach does not provide a direct measure of effectiveness. Process evaluation is easy to document and most nurses are familiar with process orientated measurement. Although process evaluation is practical, its major disadvantages are its subjectivity and inability to measure patient outcomes. Outcome evaluation focuses on the results of practice and therefore provides an objective measure of role performance and quality nursing care. A major disadvantage in using outcome evaluation is the difficulty in demonstrating that positive patient outcomes are solely attributable to specific interventions. Unless process measures are examined in relation to outcome measures, the cause of favourable and unfavourable outcome remains uncertain. Approaches being considered include measurement of patient outcomes, audit of staff training, staff wastage, ward nursing audit, self evaluation and peer review.

How will the role develop?

One exciting possibility for development of the role lies in the development of Patient Focused Care and Case Management. The CPDN could play a key role in facilitating this development by acting as leader, mentor and advisor in a multidisciplinary capacity. Influencing organizational strategy through the Clinical Leaders' Forum and other means will be increasingly important as the NHS changes begin to impact more significantly on clinical issues. Multidisciplinary teamworking will be increasingly necessary to deliver cost effective and high quality packages of care which the purchaser requires. The NHS Executive is placing an increasing emphasis on clinical effectiveness and clinical audit. The CPDN should be in an ideal position, by virtue of her experience and education, to act as leader in developing outcome indicators and clinical pathways.

The clinical research aspects of the role need to be expanded. As identified in the literature (Martin, 1990), this is one of the most neglected aspects of the CNS role and this applies to the CPDN role so far. Currently, this is due to lack of educational preparation and conflicting priorities. These issues are being addressed, as it is vital for the development of nursing that a body of knowledge continues to be built from credible clinical research and roles such as the CPDN are best placed to fulfil this.

Hamilton et al. (1990) suggest the formation of a Nursing Directorate for research and professional development, led by a director with a doctorate, an extensive background in research and experience as a CNS. The purpose of the nursing directorate is to promote the optimum level of self-care for each patient by promoting, facilitating and participating in nursing research, providing opportunities for professional growth for nursing members and providing direct care to specific patient populations. A development such as this at the RLUHT could provide the infrastructure required for research and strengthen the existing Clinical Leaders' Forum effectiveness. It would provide a strong voice and identity for nurses within the Trust to enable them to maximize their effectiveness and contribution.

The CPDN has an enormous potential contribution to make in developing nursing to face the challenges of providing better care that is value for money. Patients themselves are beginning to ask more often for personalized and efficient care and government targets are also pushing hard at traditional ways of delivering health care. This demands imaginative innovative solutions based on a thorough understanding of patients' needs. Moss Kanter (1984) believes that successful organizations are characterized by the ability of the leaders to free the powers of entrepreneurial spirit and innovation within the workforce. Individuals, she considers, have the talent to create success. Innovations are designed by individuals who develop new ideas and push for change. The CPDN, with leadership skills to think strategically, to be aware of the social and political pressures, to inspire change and support teamwork, can become the key to the success of a health care organization's strategy to thrive.

References

American Nurses Association (1976) Congress papers. In: The Scope of Nursing Practice. Description of Practice. *Clinical Nurse Spectator*, Kansas City.

Antrobus S, Whitby E (1994) New learning for the new leaders. *Nursing Management*; **1** [2]: May.

Ashurst A, Clarke D, Evitts A, Lacey J, Snashall T (1990) Creating a climate for the development of Nursing. *Nursing Practice*; **4(1)**: 18–20.

Boyd NJ, Stasiowski SA, Catoe PT, Wells PR, Marks Stahl B, Judson E, Hartman AL, Lander JH (1991) The merit and significance of clinical nurse specialists. *Journal Of Nursing Administration*; **21** [9]: 35–43.

Brieger, G, Smith, D, Meunchau, T (1989) One approach to quantifying the CNS role. *Nurse Management*; **20** [11]: 801–808.

Briggs, A (1972) *Report of the Committee on Nursing.* Department of Health & Social Security, Scottish Home & Health Department and Welsh Office. (Chairman A Briggs.)

Clay T (1987) *Nurses Power and Politics.* London: Heinemann.

Cox S (1978) The Clinical Nurse Specialist 1. The introduction of nurse specialists *Nursing Times;* July 6th: 1125.

Cumberledge Report (1986) *Neighbourhood Nursing – A Focus for Care*, Report of the Community Nursing. London: HMSO.

Department of Health (1989) *Strategy for Nursing.* London: DoH.

Department of Health (1993) *Vision for the Future.* London: DoH.

Garratt R (1987) *The Learning Organisation.* London: Fontana.

Halisbury JAH (1974) *Report of the Committee into Pay & Conditions of Service of Nurses & Midwifes.* London: DHSS, HMSO.

Ham C (1991) *The New National Health Service*. Oxford: Radcliffe Medical Press.

Hamilton L, Vincent L, Goode R, Moorhouse A, Worden RH, Jones H, Close M, Dufour S (1990) Organisational support of the clinical nurse specialist role: a nursing research and professional development directorate. *Canadian Journal of Nursing Administration*; Sep–Oct 3[3]: 9–13.

Hamric A, Spross J (eds) (1983) *The Clinical Nurse Specialist in Theory and Practice*. New York: Grune & Stratton.

Lewis EP (1970) *The Clinical Nurse Specialist*. Published by American Journal of Nursing. New York: Educational Services Division.

Loudermilk L (1990) Role ambiguity and the Clinical Nurse Specialist. *Nursing Connections*; **3** [1]: 3–11.

Martin JP (1990) Implementing the research role of the Clinical Nurse Specialist – one institution's approach. *Clinical Specialist*; **4** [3]: 1990.

Mayo A (1984) Advanced courses in Clinical Nursing: A discussion of basic assumptions and guiding principles. *American Journal of Nursing*; **44**: 579–585.

Menzies I (1960) A case study in the functioning of social systems as a defence against anxiety. *Human Relations*; **13**: 95–121.

Minter-Peglow DM, Klatt-Ellis T, Stelton S, Cutillo-Smitter T, Howard J, Wolff P (1992) Evaluation of clinical nurse specialist practice. *Clinical Nurse Specialist*; 1992 Spring **6** [1]: 28–35.

Morath JM (1988) The Clinical Nurse Specialist: evaluation issues. *Nursing Management*; **19** [3]: 72–80

Moss–Kanter R (1984) *The Change Masters*. London: Unwin.

Noll N (1987) Internal consultation as a framework for Clinical Nurse Specialist practice. *Clinical Nurse Specialist*; **1** [1]: 46–50.

Pembrey S (1991) *Guidance Paper: The Developing Role of the Clinical Practice Development Nurse*. *Oxfordshire Health Authority*.

Peplau HE (1965) *cited in* Reihl JP, McVay JE (eds) (1973) *The Clinical Nurse Specialist: Interpretations*. New York: Appleton Century Crofts.

Porter-O'Grady, T (1987) Shared governance and new organisational models. *Nursing Economics*; Nov–Dec **5** [6]: 281–286.

Prisk H (1991) The role of the Clinical Nurse Consultant and the use of research and development days. *Inforum*; **12**: 11, 13, 15.

RCN (1975) *New Horizons in Clinical Nursing*. London: RCN.

RCN (1980) *ANP/80/7 Clinical Career Structure*. London: RCN.

Salvage J (1990) The theory and practice of the new nursing. *Nursing Times Occasional Paper*; Jan 24, **86** [4]: 42–45.

Storr G (1988) The Clinical Nurse Specialist: from outside looking in. *Journal of Advanced Nursing*; **13**: 265–272.

UKCC (1990) *PREP – Post Registration Education and Practice Project*. London: UKCC.

3 Development of the lecturer/practitioner role

Pauline Stitt

In the past two decades there has been an abundance of literature on the subject of nurse education and nursing practice and where the two join forces. Within this context, the role of the Lecturer/Practitioner (L/P) has been the occasion of much debate and dissent in recent years. Individuals who have undertaken the role have shared their experiences and reported positive outcomes and benefits (Wright, 1988; Cowper, 1989; Vaughan, 1989; Guilfoyle, 1990). This chapter is concerned with these issues and critically examines the literature available, focusing upon a thematic approach in order to explore the complexity of the role. Five main themes will be addressed:

1 The historical perspective of the role, how the role originated, and the impetus for its development.
2 Role relevance in the current culture of education providers and health care providers.
3 The educational/clinical interface.
4 The paradigm shift.
5 A case study in developing the L/P role.

The historical perspective

The clinical teacher

The impetus for developing the L/P role came from the acknowledged gap between theory and practice, between what is taught in the classroom and what happens in the reality of the clinical area. Jarvis and Gibson (1985) agreed that this gap had existed ever since a separation had first been made between those who teach and those who practise.

In the 1960s an attempt was made to bridge the gap by developing the role of the clinical teacher. The irony of this role, as Davis (1989) points out, was that it made it easy for the registered nurse tutor to opt out of the clinically based aspects of the teaching curriculum. For those who have worked as clinical teachers the memory of being asked to teach students only the practical aspects of the curriculum is a sore one. The ethos of the period tended to be that clinical teachers were competent to teach practice related topics, but not what might be classed as theory. This led to an even greater divide between theory and practice.

A survey compiled by House and Sims (1976) highlighted the difficulties and lack of job satisfaction experienced by clinical teachers. This resulted in many teachers deciding to remove themselves from what was for them an intolerable situation. This they achieved by making a move in one of three directions:

- leaving formal nurse education and returning to full-time clinical work;
- going into nurse management;
- becoming a registered nurse tutor.

Although there are apparently no statistics available on the proportion of staff who followed each direction, it would appear that a large number chose to undertake a conversion course in order to become a registered tutor.

In the early 1980s the role of the clinical teacher was no longer relevant, and the last intake of students was in 1987. For some, the clinical teacher role had been seen as a stepping stone to becoming a registered nurse tutor, and was not viewed as a lifelong career move. For others it was seen as a way of combining two main aspirations – continuing to practise nursing, and at the same time educating students.

The gap left by the demise of the clinical teacher courses was filled by an abundance of conversion courses which sprang up throughout the United Kingdom. These provided the opportunity to study, often on a part-time basis, for the Certificate in Education and subsequent registration as a nurse tutor. It was argued that this was a positive move as it allowed for one level of nurse teacher (ENB, 1985). However, it removed even more teachers from the clinical area, and so the theory–practice gap widened still more (Acton et al., 1992).

One of the constraints preventing adequate practice by nurse teachers is the vexed question of staff/student ratios (SSRs). The midwifery teachers were the only ones to establish the right parameters. There is a statutory requirement for midwives to spend time in practice, and therefore an SSR of 1:10 was established to enable them to fulfil their clinical obligations (Kershaw, 1990).

There was a requirement in 1993 that all nurse teachers should spend the equivalent of 1 day per week in clinical practice. This acknowledges that organizations have to take their share of responsibility in bridging the theory–practice gap. With this in mind, both Acton et al. (1992) and the Royal College of Nursing (1993) agree that the burden cannot be shouldered by the individual alone.

The joint appointment

With the demise of the clinical teacher role came the emergence of the joint appointment. Within this role individuals owed a more than nominal allegiance to both the educational establishment and the service providers. Both the interested parties paid a proportion of the appointee's salary, and often the appointee had a contract with both.

The first joint appointment (JA) in this country was developed by Pat Ashworth and George Castledine in Manchester in 1980. Close on the heels of the Ashworth/Castledine venture came, in 1981, the joint appointment developed in Tameside by Sandra Mills and Steve Wright. These innovators of JA have acknowledged the positive aspects of the role, and its benefits in bridging the theory–practice gap. They have also sounded a note of caution regarding the cost to the individual of such an undertaking. Interestingly, one of the staunchest advocates of JA comes from the area of midwifery (Cowper, 1989). One of the reasons for the success of the venture reported by Cowper was the recognition of the need, not merely for flexibility in the role, but also for common sense and a sense of humour. How rare it is to find those qualities referred to in today's business orientated world of nurse education!

The aim of these posts was to bring together theory and practice. Wright (1983) identified four key functions of JA: teaching, nursing practice, research, and management. The assumption, according to Wright (1988) is that 'the nurse teacher can produce a climate conducive to the accomplishment of educational and practical ideals'. The expectation was that, with the provision of a more appropriate learning environment, the student would experience less of a clash between what was taught in the school of nursing and what was experienced in the practice setting. The view was that the joint appointee was in a position of sufficient authority in the clinical area to achieve this.

Literature on JA highlights authority as one of the vital features of the role. The joint appointee was expected to be in a senior position in the clinical area in order to be a change agent (Wright, 1988). A critical feature of the role was relating practices to theory and research. Significant work has been undertaken in the area of theory and practice divergence and reconciliation (Miller, 1985). The joint appointee had to undertake the role of the nurse teacher within the school of nursing. Whilst not wishing to underestimate the benefits of such a role, one cannot help but wonder whether the expectations were simply too great for any one individual to satisfy.

The post-holder not only had to juggle with clinical and educational roles, but also with a managerial role. Significant in all of this is the change agent role, and how those involved in the development of JA viewed this concept. Did the post holder have to be in charge? Did leadership have to be power-based? Could not leadership have come from the joint appointee being a role model and sharing a vision?

Those who have worked as joint appointees would be the first to acknowledge the complexity of their role and the truth that it can cause role conflict, stress, and anxiety (Ashworth and Castledine, 1980; Wright, 1988). Nevertheless, the rewards of such a role must be acknowledged also. These are identified by Lamont and Sleightholme (1989) as: 'respect from staff and students; the maintenance of clinical competence and skills; research opportunities; control over learning situations'.

If this role has been successful, why are so few joint appointees to be seen? If it has been less successful than anticipated, what is the alternative, presuming that an alternative is required to bridge the gap between theory and practice?

Role relevance of the L/P: a new breed or merely recycling?

Nurse education now uses the term L/P rather than joint appointment. Is this merely a change of name, or is it more significantly a conceptual change? What, if anything, is the difference? To those who have been involved in the development the significant factor may be the move away from focusing on the managerial and authoritative aspects of the role. This is not to imply that the L/P has no authority, but simply that the emphasis has changed. This philosophy is acknowledged by Thorne (1987) when he states: 'Management of the ward should be left to the ward sister although some exchange of role could be made to meet local circumstances'. So what is happening is a rethinking and reforming of ideas. Vickers (1983) views the L/P role as requiring a 'radical rethink of present structures and concepts'. It should not be seen merely as an adjunct to the present system, but rather, as Vaughan (1989) proposed, it must be 'taken in the context of the whole structure of practice and education'. Vaughan mentions two clearly defined aims of the L/P: to identify and maintain the standards of practice and the policies in a defined clinical area; and to prepare and contribute to the educational programme of students in relation to the theory and practice of nursing in that unit. Before discussing a definition of the role, consideration must be given to the need to develop such a role within the current climate of health care.

Among all the many contemporary changes in health and health care there are issues which exercise the minds of both providers of services and educators of nurses for the future. Two significant issues are outlined below.

The effects of the purchaser/provider split on nursing and midwifery education

Developments emerging from the Department of Health white paper (1989a) left the education of nurses in limbo. The reason for this is related to the concept of the purchaser and the provider. This concept gave a new structure to the Health Service. The professionals of the caring services could buy and offer services and expect quality, cost-effectiveness, and good patient care. This buying and selling was something new to incorporate into nurse education, and there was no earlier model to relate to. It was evident that the old paternalistic approach would disappear, and the provision of nurse education would in future be through the system of contracting. The purchasers of education would no longer 'buy' their education from the school of nursing; instead, they would think of getting value for money by 'tendering' for their contracts.

Specific educational changes

Project 2000. A New Preparation for Practice (UKCC, 1986) brought with it the requirement for links with higher education. This created the potential for an even greater gap between theory and practice.

These two issues were important enough to concentrate the mind on the roles of the two main players – the purchasers of education and the providers – and the relationship between these roles. For nurse education to keep abreast of the dynamic nature of health care, it is not enough just to visit the clinical areas now and then. There must be a significant investment in quality time spent in the clinical area. This is essential, as not only must education inform practice, but the reality of practice needs to be brought into the academic setting and inform curriculum planning. Clarity is brought to this debate by Miller (1985) commenting on the gap between theory and practice: 'Although it is clear that nursing practice must alter in order to accommodate both changes in society, and changes in our ideas about nursing, one cannot also expect practitioners to adopt idealised theories of nursing which are impossible to apply in practice'.

Is this where the L/P's strength will lie? Additionally, with this new preparation for practice, the needs of the qualified clinical staff have to be addressed. Whilst these can be met initially by workshops and discussions, there is a need for more ongoing support within the clinical setting. Also, if schools of nursing are to retain their business, they need to be responsive to the providers' requirements for education and training.

These developments were key factors in the changes required by nurse education, and were the very type to which Kanter (1990) referred in saying that the world which was external to an organization and 'poking and prodding it in numerous ways' was an important agent of change. Such considerations were not the only reasons for the development of the L/P role, but they were certainly powerful ones.

With the move of nurse education into the world of higher education, it is evident that there is a real need for the teacher of nursing to retain strong clinical contacts (Webster, 1990). It is interesting for those who have always espoused the partnership of theory and practice to observe the almost frantic efforts made to establish clinical links. The more cynical, who have moved physically from the schools of nursing within the hospital grounds into the halls of academia, will wonder why this move had not gained momentum when actually still within arm's length of the clinical area. Arguably, it is more virtuous to achieve something when the odds are stacked heavily against us.

But let us move forward in the debate in order to identify what it is we are trying to achieve. According to Davies (1989), the various amalgamations of schools/colleges of nursing with higher education are causing the role of nurse teachers to be put under the microscope. This shift into the academic world is bringing many teachers out of their comfort zone. Certain teachers may try to return to their roots and move into clinical practice again, or, as in the case of L/P, try to get the best of both worlds (Wright, 1983).

The educational/clinical interface

The L/P role must not be seen as the rejuvenation of either the clinical teacher role or the joint appointment. Whilst there are acknowledged aspects of these within the L/P role, there have to be substantial differences if the role is to be effective and not travel the rocky road of its predecessors.

The reader may find it useful to have the author's working definition of the L/P role. A lecturer practitioner is a qualified nurse with at least a first degree and with an educational/teaching qualification or ENB 998 or its equivalent. The role of the L/P is to teach within the academic environment and then integrate that theoretical teaching into practice in the clinical area. In addition, the holder of the role must work as a nurse in the clinical area and contribute to patient/client care. Complementary to the teaching and clinical facets of the role is that of staff development all of them together requiring a unified approach, as shown below:

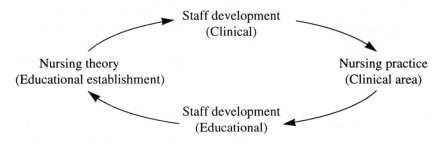

This is significantly different from the joint appointment who, as discussed earlier, tended to be in a senior position in the clinical area. In contrast to Vaughan (1989), the writer's definition does not imply that the L/P would have responsibility for the budget and skill mix, but would function as a trained member of staff and not as a ward manager. The L/P could, nevertheless, facilitate and support the ward manager in some aspects of decision making, thus taking on a significant role as a change agent. The L/P has to have authority in the clinical area, but this does not have to be of the power–coercive type (forced control), but can be of the normative–educative type (learning with education and support), as discussed by Wright (1989).

There has to be recognisable scope for the L/P to influence change. Particular areas which might benefit from the L/P's advice, support, and facilitation are: the development of policies and protocols; the development of care plans; skill mix; teaching/learning skills.

When clinical contact is established and maintained, the L/P is in a strong position to identify the changing realities of nursing and bring them to light within the theoretical aspect of the L/P's role. Therefore, there will be not only theory informing practice, but practice also nurturing theory. Such clinical practice increases the visibility of the L/P to health care providers (Lamont and Sleightholme, 1989).

It has long been acknowledged that educators must consistently make their presence felt in the clinical area and earn high credibility among the staff with whom they work (Polifroni and Schmalenberg, 1985). This is one of the most important aspects of the L/P role, and one which it takes skill and commitment to achieve, particularly the skill to move quickly from one mode of thinking to another.

What must not be overlooked is the actual benefit this role brings to the relationship between clinical providers and the educational establishment. It enables reciprocity of ideas to become a reality, and it allows for open, frank discussions based upon mutual respect and interest. In addition, the potential for identifying and exploring research interests is enhanced.

The L/P role can be seen to have a value in that it contributes to developing the body of knowledge of the nursing profession. Significantly, it makes more appropriate use of research findings within clinical practice. With the move of health care and therefore health care education into the market place, the need for each to know the other's business is of paramount importance. Within this market place it is only those who can identify the business opportunities who can survive.

The paradigm shift

'Paradigms are examples or patterns on which practice can be developed'. They can be seen as providing a broad range of perspectives on nursing in order to provide information for practice (England, 1989).

The individual who intends to undertake the L/P role has to make a significant conceptual leap. The paradigm shift is not a once and for all shift, but a constant pendular movement between the clinical model and that of the academic world. In an ideal world there would be no need for this oscillation, as the two would integrate. What the L/P has to achieve is an ideal encompassing all aspects of the role. This cannot be achieved immediately, as for too long the organizational restraints of nurse education have allowed a denial of such a need. In the current climate of health care such a paradigm shift should be acknowledged as not only desirable but essential.

Case study: developing the L/P role

When two amalgamated schools of nursing and midwifery were integrated into higher education in Liverpool there was an immediate impact which was not anticipated. This was the perception of providers of health care that they had been abandoned by education, or at least, if the links had not been broken, they had been severely strained.

The new school recognized the potential conflicts to which this situation could give rise, and to address the problem the role of the link teacher was developed. This provided the clinical areas used for training with a named teacher who had a multi-faceted role as resourcer, facilitator, communicator, teacher, advocate, and supporter. This role continues, although the nature of the school and the internal demands made on the staff result in the staff being able to spend only a half to one day in the role.

It was recognized that the changing nature of the school and the provider units necessitated the development of a higher profile for some roles; thus, discussions were started about developing the role of the L/P. A small working group was set up, consisting of academic staff and clinical managers to consider the parameters of the L/P role, as perceived by the school and the provider units. At this stage it was agreed that it would be difficult to draw up a job specification, since that would have to be different for every role. Instead, Liverpool JMU agreed to draw up initially a person specification, as shown below:

Table 3.1   Person specification

The applicant for an L/P post must have:

Attainments
- First level nurse
- A relevant first degree
- A teaching qualification or ENB 998
- A minimum of 2 years' clinical experience (in the appropriate field)
- Hold a certificate for Advanced/Higher Technology Nursing (where appropriate, for example ICU, CCU, A and E)

Aptitudes
- Motivator
- Facilitator
- Communicator
- Exceptional time management skills
- Excellent interpersonal skills
- Resourceful

Disposition
- Approachable
- Open
- Trustworthy
- Loyal
- Sense of humour

Intelligence and interests
- Creative
- Visionary
- Customer awareness
- Quality initiatives
- Commitment to both pre- and post-registration education
- Practice based research
- Staff development

Whilst it was acknowledged that it was going to be difficult to find such a paragon, it was felt that to go for less would undervalue the role and consequently the right applicants would be dissuaded from coming forward.

Following this thumbnail sketch of the attributes needed in an L/P, a job specification was also now seen to be necessary. Unlike Vaughan (1989) and others who have undertaken this role, this individual is not seen as someone to take on the role of the ward manager, but rather as someone who would begin to build bridges between education and practice. One important area to focus on is that of vocabulary and communication. Miller (1985) observes that theorists tend to use complicated and obscure language with reference to concepts which are unfamiliar to the average nurse. The L/P could help to demystify the language. The principal responsibilities are identified in Table 3.2.

Table 3.2   Principal responsibilities of L/P (as defined by Liverpool JMU)

Academic
- Ensure a high standard of academic and professional practice experience for students.
- Lead in the preparation of clinical staff as mentors and assessors within a specified area of practice.
- Liaise with individual personal tutors in providing tutorial support to a group of students.
- Act and participate as an associate course/module leader where requested.
- Participate in student assessments.
- Lead in the monitoring of clinical placements within the school's agreed framework.
- Promote research awareness and informed clinical practice with students and qualified practitioners.
- Be responsible for own professional development.

Clinical
- Undertake a minimum of one clinical shift per week which includes a patient/client caseload.
- Assist and support all clinical nurses in the ward/department/community to develop clinical practice.
- Develop and set clinical nursing policies.
- Participate in and facilitate clinical research and identify potential areas for research.
- Resource clinical staff in terms of orientation and development needs.

In addition, subject discipline, managerial/administrative, and personal responsibilities were included.

Following this interpretation of the L/P role, the next agenda item was convincing others of the benefits of the role. Whilst many clinical and academic colleagues agreed in principle with the concept of the role, they were yet to be convinced of its benefits. It was important to persuade all sides, since there was a cost implication. This cost was salary, as both partners would need to contribute to the L/P pay. In today's climate, cost is a major issue as no one has any money to spare. The cost benefit of the role can be seen below:

- Development of students who are ultimately better prepared to practise, owing to the lessening of the gap between theory and practice.
- Benefits of someone who is highly qualified and has retained clinical working skills by working in the clinical area.
- Staff development. Clinical staff exposed regularly to someone who has access to higher education and can therefore contribute to their development.
- Positive communication link between school and health care providers.
- Someone available to implement research findings and act as a change agent in the clinical area.
- Keeping the school aware of changes and developments in clinical practice which can bring the reality aspect into teaching.
- Enabling academics to contextualize practice, seeing it where it happens and

therefore heightening their appreciation of a clinical staff's difficulties in putting some of nursing theory into practice.

This work resulted in a paper being sent to all clinical managers (directors of nursing or equivalent) to ascertain if there would be any interest in the development of the role both now and in the future. The majority of clinical managers took a positive view of the role, whilst they were at this stage not ready to commit any resources to it.

The author was approached by one directorate nursing manager to develop the role within the intensive care unit. At this point the parameters of the role had not been defined. It was thought that developing the role would provide a useful pilot study.

Time span for development of role

It was evident that a great deal of planning had to be invested in the development. The issues that had to be addressed were:

- Aims and objectives of role.
- Negotiation with clinical managers.
- Designing contracts.
- Designing person specifications.
- Designing role specifications.
- Interviewing potential staff for the role.
- Orientation of staff.
- Supporting the L/P.

In total, it took approximately 6–8 months to establish the first role between the school of health care and the provider unit. As the role was evolving it was agreed to establish it on a 1-year fixed term contract.

The person appointed to the role was a senior lecturer who was course leader for the ENB course 920 intensive care course. Because of unforeseen circumstances regarding course management difficulties, the role itself only lasted for 6 months. During this time, it was evident that the role was beneficial to all parties. The was because the senior lecturer, who managed and taught on course 920, was able to follow the students through to the practice area and evaluate the effectiveness of the theory taught in the reality of practice. It kept the senior lecturer cognizant of changes and developments as they occurred in practice. Not insignificantly, the senior lecturer was able to identify the professional development needs in the intensive care unit and provide for some of these himself. Where this was not possible, the nurse manager was kept informed of the staff's development needs.

The fact that this role was short-lived has not been a deterrent to the development of future posts, either in intensive care or in other areas. The evaluation of the role was positive and enthusiasm was generated to do more to attract interest in such initiatives.

The next initiative involved a clinical practitioner from a training ward in one of the Liverpool hospitals being brought into an L/P post, again on a short-term contract. What was encouraging about this post was that it espoused further the concept of partnership between the school and the health care providers. That is, the school was as willing to attract clinicians into the academic setting as to place lecturers into the clinical environment. The L/P's contract has been completed at the time of writing.

The post holder of the above role set the following objectives to try to ensure that both educational and clinical commitments were attended to (Thain, 1993):

Educational objectives

1 Identify possible areas of input and circulate these to the teaching staff.
2 Consolidate and expand lecturing skills, to cover a wider range of subjects.
3 Gain abilities in leading small groups acting as facilitator of discussions etc.
4 Liaise with placement areas regarding students' performance.
5 Maintain contact with students on placements.
6 Participate in the marking of students' assignments, with critical evaluation of skills.
7 Participate in curriculum development within the Common Foundation Programme.
8 Participate in standard setting for the Common Foundation Programme.
9 Maintain research input.
10 Act as a role model within the clinical setting.

Clinical objectives

1 Provide expert senior nurse support for bone marrow transplant (BMT) unit.
2 Provide input to the development of the new BMT unit, and encourage and support other staff in the identification and development of new ideas in this area.
3 Participate in standard setting and monitoring in the BMT unit and the ward.
4 Develop learning material for students and qualified staff and promote its use.
5 Develop a resource base for use by all staff.
6 Provide support to mentors and assessors, and act as mentor for a number of staff.
7 Work as primary nurse within the BMT unit.
8 Plan and organize study days, in conjunction with other ward staff, on appropriate subjects.
9 Identify research opportunities for self, and assist and encourage other staff to do the same.

While these objectives may seem to be well balanced, the reality turned out to be a little different (Thain, 1993). One of the L/P's main aims was the development of teaching skills and learning strategies. The main concern after 6 months was that too much emphasis was placed on the academic part of the role, and this consequently reduced the impact on the clinical role. There was dissonance between the students on the ward and those in the classroom. Learning materials, in the form of teaching packages for students and for clinical staff, were developed in the clinical area. In an ideal situation the L/P should follow the students through to the clinical area; however, some compromises had to be made in an effort to establish the role. While not achieving all the objectives as comprehensively as expected, the L/P would like to see the role continue. This has to be seen as a positive development (Thain, 1993).

This informal evaluation has provided some guidance for future strategies in the development of the role. Nevertheless, the last two L/P posts to emerge have been very different. The first, which is between the private sector and the school, illustrates the shifting nature of health care. It recognizes the need for both practitioner and educators to be open-minded about where health and social policies are leading. This development provides the opportunity to bring some of the business of the private sector into the school, and raise the awareness of both students and staff to the many challenges within health care today.

Consideration must be given to the fact that some 30 000 nurses are employed in the private sector and their education and development needs have to be met (Holloway, 1990). In addition, the private provider is the recipient of all the previously mentioned benefits and advantages of the role.

The second post has a three-dimensional focus, as it is formed between a local community (NHS) trust and family health service authority and the school. This tripartite relationship means that the post holder functions as a district nurse, a practice nurse, and a lecturer. Whilst it is not certain that it is the first of its kind in the country, it is unlikely that there are many such innovations.

With the impact of Care in the Community (DOH, 1989b) now being strongly felt, this complex and extremely demanding role provides a unique opportunity for the post holder to influence practice in various community settings. There is also the opportunity not merely to bridge the gap between theory and practice, but to contribute via student education, to be at the interface between hospital and community and so impact on the move towards a 'seamless service'.

These two roles are in the early stages of development, and it is too soon to evaluate them. A careful monitoring of the role is being maintained throughout the period of tenure, and there is to be a formal evaluation before the final date of the contract.

One of the most significant aspects of the two developments is that the post holders, who had permanent contracts in their previous posts, were willing to take a risk and go onto a fixed term contract. The reasons for this are complex, but two of the most important are: the individual's desire and enthusiasm for such a role; and the perception that it is a prestigious role to undertake in terms of professional development.

Evaluating the L/P role. The way forward

It appears that there is a great deal of energy expended in the development and implementation of L/P posts. Therefore those who take on these roles must have a vision of the rewards for putting themselves into what can only be seen as a complex, demanding, and at times draining role. One of the most immediate rewards is that of improved quality. Part of the L/P's role is in the process of educating the knowledgeable doer for the future, and ultimately this leads to improved patient care. Improved patient care leads to improved outcomes and an increase in patient satisfaction. Improved quality of care could also lead to earlier discharge, which would make the role very cost effective.

The follow scenarios show the kind of thing that can happen.

The L/P has taught students about the importance of information and communication in reducing anxiety before surgery. All the relevant research is used as evidence for this, and the student follows the L/P's example. Patients are better informed before surgery, and they are therefore likely to require less post operative analgesia. Cost effectiveness is achieved.

The L/P alerts the clinical staff to research on various aspects of wound dressings, new techniques, and infection control. The implementation by the clinical staff of such research findings results in a reduction in infection, a reduced length of stay for patients, fewer investigations, less medication, and increased patient satisfaction.

The L/P is able to identify specific staff development needs and is able to meet some of these in-house, which means reduced cost in terms of study days and possibly staff replacement. Alternatively, the L/P directs and advises staff on the most appropriate ways of meeting their development needs. Thus the needs can be met in an appropriate and cost effective way.

There is no suggestion in what I have said above that such things could not happen without an L/P, but with all the many demands on the clinical staff they are simply less likely to happen.

The greatest measure of the success of the L/P role would be if eventually there were no need for such a specific role, with every qualified nurse taking on the role as a matter of course.

References

Acton L, Gough P, McCormack B, Charlesworth G, Kanneh A, Masterson A (1992) The clinical nurse tutor debate. Clinical credibility and expertise for nurse teachers. *Nursing Times*; **88 (32)**: 38–41.

Ashworth PM, Castledine G (1980) Joint service-education appointments in nursing. *Medical Teacher*; **2**: 295–299.

Cowper A (1989) The joint appointment that works. *Midwife, Health Visitor, and Community Nurse*; **25** [10]: 420–422.

Davies J (1989) Who or what are lecturer/practitioners? *Senior Nurse*; **9** [10]: 22.

Department of Health (1989a) *Working for Patients. The White Paper*. London: HMSO.

Department of Health (1989b) *Caring for People: Community Care in the Next Decade and Beyond*. London: HMSO.

England M (1989) Nursing diagnosis. A conceptual framework. In: Fitzpatrick JK, Whall AL (eds), *Conceptual Models of Nursing. Analysis and Application*. California: Appelton and Large, pp 347–369.

English National Board (1985) *Professional Education/Training Courses*. Consultation paper ENB.

Guilfoyle JF (1990) Responding to a human need. Lecturer/practitioner in human sexuality. *Professional Nurse*; 6 [1]: 33–6.

Holloway B (1990) Public and private co-operation. *Nursing*; 4 [10]: 21–23.

House V, Sims A (1976) Teachers of nursing in the United Kingdom. A description of their cultures. *Journal of Advanced Nursing*; 1, 495–505.

Jarvis P, Gibson S (1985) *The Teacher Practitioner in Nursing, Midwifery, and Health Visiting*. London: Croom Helm.

Kanter RM (1990) *The Change Masters*. London: Unwin Hyman.

Kershaw B (1990) Clinical credibility and nurse teachers. *Nursing Standard*; 4 [51]: 46–47.

Lamont R, Sleightholme C (1989) Nursing faculty and clinical practice. *The Canadian Nurse*; 85 (8), 22–25.

Miller A (1985) The relationship between nursing theory and nursing practice. *Journal of Advanced Nursing*; 10: 417–424.

Polifroni EC, Schmalenberg C (1985) Faculty practice that works: two examples. *Nursing Outlook*; 33 (5): 226–228.

Royal College of Nursing (1993): *Teaching in the New World*. London: RCN.

Thain C (1993) *The Role of the Lecturer/Practitioner*. Unpublished.

Thorne T (1987) Clinical credibility. *Senior Nurse*; 6 [5]: 29.

United Kingdom Central Council (1986) *Project 2000. A New Preparation for Practice*. London: UKCC.

Vaughan B (1989) Two roles – one job. Lecturer practitioner to bridge the theory–practice gap in nurse education. *Nursing Times*; 85 [11]: 52.

Vickers G (1983) *The Art of Judgement*. London: Harper & Row.

Webster R (1990) The role of the nurse teachers. *Senior Nurse*; 10 [8]: 6–8.

Wright S (1983) Joint appointments. The best of both worlds? *Nursing Times*; 79 [42]: 25–9.

Wright S (1988) Joint appointments: handle with care. Combining a clinical post with teaching. *Nursing Times*; 84 [1]: 32–3.

Wright S (1989) *Changing Nursing Practice*. London: Edward Arnold.

4 Development of the role of the rheumatology nurse practitioner

Stella O'Gorman

Change is not made without inconvenience, even from worse to better.

Samuel Johnson (1709–1784)

This chapter will take the reader through a series of experiences which could ultimately be used to improve quality of care for rheumatic patients. It was a voyage of discovery, originating from the recognition that patients attending a rheumatology clinic received very little specialist help from the nursing staff in the outpatient department. This lack of support was not intentional, but stemmed from nurses having insufficient knowledge to bring about improvements in care. This lack of knowledge was due to nursing staff being content to support the medical model and maintain a comfortable *status quo*. This was coupled with a management ethos which was unable or unwilling to encourage and support the necessary staff development. It was and remains a very uncomfortable journey at times.

The nursing profession is undergoing important changes with the advent of Project 2000 and the implementation of recent Department of Health reports: *Working for Patients* (1989), *Caring for People* (1989a), *Strategy for Nursing*, (1989c), *Research for Health*, (1991, 1993b) and *Vision for the Future* (1993a). Schober (1993) tells us that nurses hold the key to caring relationships at a time when people are at their most vulnerable. Moreover Lo Bindo-Wood and Haber (1986) make it clear that we are now accountable for quality of client care. However, such themes are often met with varying degrees of inertia at the grassroots of practice. Even now, nurses still question their own reasons and motives for attempting to bring about changes when colleagues and other professionals seem opposed to the new ideas. Salvage (1985) firmly believes that we must ally ourselves with the patients and continue to 'speak their language and promote their interests'.

Rheumatology – a specialism

The difficulty nurses have in bringing about change is, in many ways, epitomized in the speciality of rheumatology. Although approximately 250 diseases (Wood, 1986) come under the title of rheumatology, as a specialist subject in its own right, it is a comparative newcomer. Twenty years ago, patients with arthritis would probably see either the general physician or an orthopaedic surgeon. Their chances of having a nurse qualified in rheumatic diseases would be even more remote and probably confined to the specialist spa centres dotted around the country.

This position has continued until recently, despite 10 million people having arthritis in the UK. Gutch and Cope (1992) give a number of interesting statistics. One million of the people with arthritic conditions are under 45, 23% between 45 and 64 and 41% of those who are 65 years or older experience the condition. Arthritis also accounts for 11% of all working days lost – approximately 69 million working days per year and an estimated productivity loss of £1 billion. The cost of arthritis to the National Health Service was estimated at nearly £500 million in 1989 and because of demographic changes, this is expected to increase by 14% by 2001. It therefore seems even more extraordinary that in the government's consultative document, *Health of the Nation* (1992), arthritis was not included in the key health areas to be considered.

The rheumatology nurse – researching the role

As the result of the award of a local scholarship, the opportunity to look at the role of the rheumatology nurse and how that could be developed became available. Help was sought from two of the pioneers in rheumatology nursing in this country – Vicky Stephenson and Sally Chesson. Stephenson and Chesson founded the Royal College of Nursing Rheumatology Forum over 10 years ago and the former was awarded an RCN Fellowship in 1987 for her valuable work in rheumatology. The programme proposed by them included visits to hospitals in six regions in this country and three in Sweden. The visits were planned with the idea of gaining as much knowledge and experience as possible from a variety of hospitals. Rheumatology patients are cared for in very different setting, and the manner in which that care is organized and the priorities each hospital decides can influence the delivery of nursing care.

Summary of the visits

The facilities

Service and facilities for rheumatic patients vary enormously from region to region in this country and in Sweden. In Sweden, for example, all three hospitals in this report had an out-patients department, a conventional 7-day ward, a 5-day ward and departments devoted entirely to the care of the rheumatic patient. Two also had day wards and one, a ward for the care of patients receiving mud treatments. It was not unusual for the state to pay for patients to go to spa centres abroad for several weeks rest and treatment. The advent of trusts and competitive tendering has made it more and more impossible for those hospitals established close to England's historic spa resorts to survive. Conversely, spa centres in Germany, Sweden and Spain have developed and prospered.

In England, the best facilities were in a recently opened purpose-built unit. Not only did this have the latest equipment, but had also considered accommodation for the rest of the multidisciplinary team involved in the care of rheumatic patients.

A purpose-built unit is the ideal, but most hospitals need to make the best of what they have. Five hospitals were in refurbished premises that fulfilled the needs of the patients reasonably well.

A hospital in one of the London districts faced great problems, with services scattered between three hospitals, all with outdated, cramped accommodation, and the added problems of travel and transport in a large city. Understandably, community services for rheumatic patients had been developed rapidly to cope with these special problems.

Towards specialized care

In all the hospitals there was a deep sense of caring for and involvement with the patients. However, some hospitals were far more advanced than others in establishing the care of the rheumatoid patient as a speciality of its own. Here, one found innovation, forward thinking, good communication, research and patients who were empowered to take control of their own disease. These departments were open to change and were always seeking better methods of managing the treatment and care of their patients. The quality of care was so obviously superior.

Four aspects of the data collected were analysed and compared:

1 The total number of population served (Fig. 4.1).
2 The total number of consultants in each unit (Fig. 4.2).
3 The total number of rheumatology nurses – sisters + grades above (Fig. 4.3).
4 Criteria used to evaluate nursing input (Fig. 4.4).

Each aspect is summarized in a block diagram. In the first diagram, the hospitals are listed in order of population served. For ease of comparison they are listed in the same order in the following three diagrams. The parent hospital is included for comparison.

All population figures in England were based on those in the *Hospital Year Book* of 1990. The figures for (1) were difficult to assess. It was a regional unit, which also took patients from many areas throughout the country. However, to say they served a population of over 50 million, or even the 3 million in the region, would seem to be an exaggeration and an impossibility with a possible in-patient intake of 50. Therefore, the figures for (1) had to be an estimation.

The regional units of (1) and (2) had very active research units and therefore had the largest establishments of consultants. However, the real signs of the inequalities in the NHS do seem to be proved when the consultant establishment for (3), which served a district population of almost 550 000, was just one.

Sweden has managed to achieve the enviable position of providing a

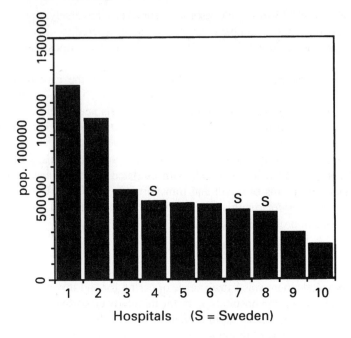

Figure 4.1   Total number of population served

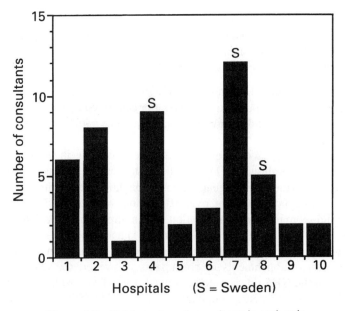

Figure 4.2   Total number of consultants in each unit

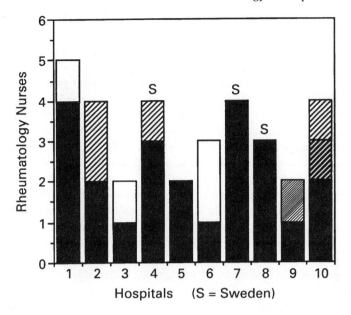

Figure 4.3   Number of rheumatology nurses, sisters and grades above.
■ Sister; ▨ Nurse consultant; ▨ Nurse specialist; ▨ Nurse practitioner;
□ Metrologist.

1   Primary nursing.

2   Nurse-run clinics.

3   Patient assessment.

4   Patient education.

5   Multidisciplinary education classes.

6   Multidisciplinary team meetings.

7   Patient self-administration of drugs.

8   Nurse practitioner clinics.

9   Research.

Figure 4.4   Criteria used to evaluate nursing output

rheumatology specialist for 40 000 of the population; England continues to struggle with an approximately 1–400 000 ratio.

Sweden's consultant establishments were difficult to assess, but these were the figures given in each of the hospital's lists and confirmed by members of the senior staff. There does not seem to be the exact equivalent post in Sweden, but all the doctors included in the figures were senior specialists.

At the moment, a great deal of confusion exists with regard to titles used by nurses who have specialist knowledge of rheumatology. Some would say that a ward sister in charge of a rheumatology ward is, in fact, a nurse specialist, that a nurse advising at hospital level is a nurse practitioner and that a senior nurse who gives advice at district or regional level is a nurse consultant. However, the UKCC (1993) seems to prefer to link titles to academic qualification and advocate two levels of senior clinical nurse – specialist nurse and advanced practitioner. The advanced practitioner would be expected to be at least at Masters degree level. Many nurses throw up their hands in horror at this latest proposal thinking that advanced practitioner posts will be filled with academic geniuses who have few practical skills and are unable to relate to the patients. It could also be argued that, in some instances, nurses are appointed to these crucial roles with insufficient experience and knowledge and unfortunately do more harm than good (Powe, 1993). Add to this list, metrologist (one who collects measurement data), research nurse and liaison nurse and the picture becomes even more confusing.

In this critique, nurses from sister level and above were included following the assumption that senior nurses are responsible for creating the ethos of a department. Only G grade sisters were included, apart from one F grade sister who was in charge of a ward area. The titles are those used by the individual hospitals.

Criteria used to evaluate nursing input

Deciding which criteria could be used to evaluate the nurse's role proved difficult. In the end, it became a personal decision, although backed up by research articles, observations of modern trends and a consensus of opinion of the leading rheumatology nurses in England and the USA. They were not put forward as standards by which all rheumatology units should be judged now and forever more. At the time, it was a way of assessing whether or not nurses were seeking to update and develop their practice. It was a way of finding out whether or not nurses were including methods which have been developed specifically to improve the care of the rheumatology patient. It was a useful yardstick and can be adapted and updated as research changes and influences practice.

The nine criteria (Fig. 4.4) are seen by authors such as Bird et al. (1985) and Pigg et al. (1985) as being the way forward envisaged in the government White Paper, *Working for Patients* (1989a). They will 'enable a higher quality of patient care to be obtained from the resources which the nation is able to devote to the NHS'.

The hospitals in the survey received a point for each of the criteria found to be part of nursing practice (Fig. 4.5).

Primary nursing	*	*		*				*		*
Nurse run clinics		*		*		*	*	*	*	*
Patient assessment	*	*	*			*				*
Patient education	*	*	*	*		*		*	*	*
Team education		*		*			*	*	*	
Team meetings		*	*	*	*		*	*	*	*
Self-medication										*
Practitioner clinics		*		*					*	*
Nursing research		*		*				*		*
Total	3	8	3	7	1	3	3	6	5	8
Hospitals (S = Sweden)	1	2	3	S4	5	6	S7	S8	9	10

Figure 4.5   Evaluation criteria – points scored as *

Justification for the criteria used for evaluation

Primary nursing

The concept of primary nursing originated in America. It was first described by Manthey et al. in 1970. The concept emerged from concern about the fragmentation of patient care in the hospital setting. An organizational pattern was developed which enabled each nurse to take continuous responsibility for the total nursing care of between three and six patients. Since then, primary nursing has had a chequered career, certainly in this country, probably due to the lack of dedication which is required by management and nursing staff to bring about its implementation (Farmer, 1986). Nevertheless, those nurses who have embraced this approach agree that both patient care and staff satisfaction are greatly enhanced by its introduction. Hegyvary (1982) in America and Pearson (1988), in this country, reported that results of primary nursing projects indicated that patients and their families expressed more confidence in the nursing care. There was significantly higher patient satisfaction and patients were more socially active where primary nursing ideas were incorporated into practice. Bond (1993) states that primary nursing put the patient at the forefront of care and raised the status of clinical nursing.

The Patients' Charter (1991) included in its recommendations that each patient should have the right to receive the care of a named nurse, midwife or health visitor. The General Secretary of the RCN, Christine Hancock, agreed that the named nurse found its clearest expression in primary nursing, but conceded that, at that time, it was practised in only 16% of acute hospital settings.

Pigg (1989) states that the nurse caring for the arthritic patient has a primary role in co-ordinating the activities, instructions and orders of other care providers into the patient's life style and that this co-ordination is patient centred. Hill (1985) found that patients responded to seeing the same nurse at each outpatient appointment and that the supportive nursing approach to chronic illness resulted in a better patient outcome.

Five hospitals in this survey had implemented primary nursing with varying degrees of success. All agreed that it brought about a closer personal contact with the patient and his family and created a therapeutic environment in which healing could take place.

Nurse-run clinics

Many drug monitoring clinics are now being run by nurses, independent of the medical staff in hospital and the community. Protocols are drawn up and agreed with the doctors concerned. Patients on secondline drugs, such as gold and sulphasalazine, receive care, education and advice from nurses on most of their visits to the hospital or general practitioner. They see the doctor only occasionally when problems requiring medical advice arise. *The Strategy for Nursing*, 1989, encouraged nurses to develop an independent role and agreed that 'observing signs, symptoms and reactions, carrying out appropriate intervention prescribed by nurses themselves, together with accurate and full reporting and recording, represents specific nursing functions which complement the equally specific diagnostic and prescribing skills of the doctor'. Visits to a clinic for regular blood checks, which these drugs require, also provides a valuable opportunity for patients to share problems with staff. It is, therefore, important that these nurses should be qualified, well informed and given the opportunity to update their education.

All units caring for arthritic patients, because of the modern belief that the disease should be treated aggressively to minimize joint damage, are involved in drug monitoring (Bird et al., 1985). Some consultants refer most of their patients back to the general practitioner for monitoring, others prefer to monitor all their patients themselves with or without the help of the nursing staff.

Patients who need to take medication on a long-term basis do need support and encouragement over long periods of time. Jette (1982) found that there was a need to ensure patient compliance in order to evaluate treatment efficacy. Neuberger (1984) felt that the nurse has the knowledge and skills necessary to effectively monitor medication.

In seven of the hospitals visited, nurses had a definite role to play in the drug monitoring clinics.

Patient assessment

Bird et al. (1985) acknowledge that access to serial assessments of the patient's progress, over a period of time, will be of great value to the clinicians in deciding which type of drug to administer or what surgical procedure to employ in order to arrest the advance of the arthritis or to improve function. Pigg (1985) argues that the nursing assessment of the patient with a rheumatic condition provides the basis for nursing diagnosis and intervention, as well as data that supplement the information gathered by other care providers.

Oldham et al. (1992) argue that it is no longer acceptable for nurses to use subjective methods of assessing their patients if valid measurement tools are available. Remarks such as 'seems to have improved' or 'is coping better with activities of daily living' are not acceptable when attempting functional assessment. Bowling (1991) confirms that for the speciality of rheumatology, there are numerous methods of measuring functional disability and health status, all of which have been rigorously tested for reliability and validity. Most of them are easy to use and to score, many are used by the medical profession and drug firms to assess patients' health status. Such methods include the Ritchie Articular Index (Ritchie et al., 1968), visual analogue scales for pain, as well as grip strength scores and the recording of early morning stiffness duration. Unfortunately, as Pagana and Pagana (1982) found with many acceptable measurement tools, few are used routinely by nurses.

In five of the hospitals nurses were using these methods of assessment.

Patient education

Le Gallez (1984) found that to help and encourage self-management, patients with chronic illness need to be given detailed information about their disease and that this patient education should be an integral part of total patient care. The Patients' Charter reiterates that the patient has a right to be given a clear explanation of any treatment proposed, including any risks and any alternatives, before deciding whether or not to agree to treatment. Chesson (1984) confirms that as nurses have close and continuing contact with patients they are in an excellent position to teach, counsel and support.

There is no shortage of educational material for nurses to give to patients with rheumatic disease. The Arthritis and Rheumatism Council (ARC) and Arthritis Care (AC) produce an excellent range of booklets and information sheets which will answer most questions concerning day to day management. There are numerous specialist organizations such as Lupus UK, Raynaud's Association, British Sjogrens Society and many others all of which produce information leaflets usually free of charge. Many hospitals develop their own leaflets, particularly on information for patients receiving secondline drug therapy.

Giving out information leaflets is an improvement on giving no information at all, but patient education also requires time to assess the requirements of the individual, provide relevant information and evaluate outcomes.

In seven of the hospitals, nurses were actively promoting patient education.

Multidisciplinary education classes

In confirming treatment of arthritic patients as a multidisciplinary responsibility, Pigg (1989) promotes education as an important element in management and a major independent responsibility of all health professionals. In seeking to employ a multidisciplinary approach to education, Althoff and Nordenskiold (1985) suggest that rheumatoid arthritis is a complex disease and that joint protection is an important element in its control. In their teaching programme on joint protection they stress the importance of including the cognizance of other disciplines to reinforce instructions, to maintain the cross-fertilization of ideas between staff members and to make sure that the patient's individual needs are being considered.

For many years, the multidisciplinary team approach to patient education has been recognized as an excellent method of bringing together the expertise of the team for the benefit of the rheumatic patient. Usually, the education classes take the form of a series of sessions, each one devoted to a topic and led by the expert in that subject. The patients can either be inpatients or outpatients and usually attend one class a week lasting for about 2 h. The classes can be in the form of a rolling programme, each programme lasting from six to eight sessions. There is no shortage of topics for such meetings and these can range from disease process, joint protection and drug therapy to social benefits and complementary therapy. Lorig and Fries (1993) acknowledge the need for team members to impart knowledge to the patients, but also emphasize that this is in order that the individual can be the best judge of which self management techniques suit them best. Programmes should, in these days of patient-centred care, be constantly evaluated and updated for and by the patients themselves.

Education classes took place in five of the hospitals in this survey.

Multidisciplinary team meetings

Wright (1982) argues that the concept of team approach with each discipline supplying special, yet overlapping skills is accepted in principle although not always in practice!

Care of the rheumatic patient requires input from several professional disciplines. Doctors, nurses, physiotherapists, occupational therapists and social workers all have an important part to play in the care of these patients. It is vitally important that they communicate with each other, on equal terms, to share knowledge and information and to prevent overlap of treatment.

Many hospitals claim to have multidisciplinary team meetings. Further questioning reveals that meetings rarely take place, disagreements have arisen amongst team members and only some attend or, as in one hospital in this survey, the team meetings consisted of the doctor and the physiotherapists.

Another hospital claimed to have meetings every morning on the ward, but one understandably confused student occupational therapist reported that the rest of the day was spent in arguing who should treat the patient next! Sadly the nurse was often the missing team member, the reasons given being pressure of work and lack of staff.

Patients who have suffered from rheumatic disease appreciate the need for an organized team approach. Ann Macfarlane (1985), chairman of the London Regional Committee of Arthritis Care and a victim of Still's disease at the age of 4 years, understood the need for good team communication and during her long stays in hospital had many opportunities to observe the 'team' approach. She felt that a long-standing condition could disable not just the person who has it, but also those who come into constant contact with such patients. She reiterated the need for members of the multidisciplinary team to communicate, work closely with and support each other. She had witnessed rivalry and jealousy between professional staff and had seen the fear and insecurity that it could generate amongst patients. Pigg (1985) argues that, in most multidisciplinary team settings, the patient's physician is the designated leader of the team, but the role of the team co-ordinator could fall to any member. She takes the position that the nurse's role in the team may vary, but she has a primary responsibility to ensure that each patient is involved and participates in a comprehensive management programme.

Eight hospitals scored a point for organizing team meetings.

Patient self-administration of drugs (PSAD)

PSAD is becoming the policy for many hospitals. MacDonald and MacDonald (1982) conceded that many patients in the past, on discharge from hospital, have gone home and been faced with an array of bottles, the contents of which have been completely unknown to them. This led to overdosage, underdosage and dissatisfaction with their treatment.

Pigg (1985) asserts that the patient who is responsible for his or her medication at home should be able to manage it whilst he or she is in hospital. Those with chronic rheumatic disease have had many years of learning coping strategies, including when to take their medication with greatest effect for them. Nothing can be more soul destroying for a patient than to have to wait for the timed arrival of the drug trolley in order to be given two simple pain killers which are readily available at home and which most people keep in their handbags or pockets. Newly diagnosed patients need to learn about their own individual drug management – what works best for them. Surely the best place for them to learn is whilst they have expert help and supervision in hospital.

One hospital was involved in a PSAD programme; two were looking at ways of implementing the scheme. One nurse practitioner had tried to establish the practice on the ward, but failed because of nursing staff opposition.

Nurse practitioner clinics

The role of the nurse practitioner has been accepted in certain areas for many years. Stoma care, Diabetic and MacMillan nurses are able to work autonomously and patient care has been enhanced by their expertise. Bird et al. (1985) acknowledged that nurse practitioners or equivalent were being used extensively in the United States in the provision of health care programmes for patients with chronic medical complaints such as arthritis. He felt that the British system could be improved by a comparable provision of such health professionals.

Marsden (1992), discussing the NHS Management Executive's report of 1990 and the National Audit Office's 1991 report (HMSO, 1991), stated that outpatient nurses needed to adapt to survive. They needed to find ways of developing and promoting clinical excellence in outpatient nursing. He felt that specialist outpatient nurses might be able to complement outpatient services already available from hospital doctors, adding depth and breadth to the services that providers have to offer. In particular, they had a leading role to play in health promotion.

Developing the role of the nurse practitioner can meet with opposition from doctors who feel threatened by nursing innovation. In 1983, the Chairman of the British Medical Association's Central Committee for Hospital Medical Services wrote, 'I think my chaps are worried that some people in nursing see the nurse's role as one which can exercise its own authority independently of the medical role. It is these suggestions, that medicine and nursing can be operating in parallel but not necessarily pursuing the same objectives, that make doctors uneasy'. Rafferty (1986), however, urged nurses to be seen to make a positive, practical and thoughtful contribution to patient care and felt that this would reap its own rewards. Fenton (1985) expected the clinical nurse specialist to be an expert in the delivery of advanced nursing care, systems analysis, change strategy, as well as giving situational and emotional support for nursing staff.

Where rheumatology nurse practitioner roles were accepted, their work was much appreciated by all members of the multidisciplinary team. Moreover, these nurses worked well with the doctors, relieving them of the counselling, education, routine assessments and the ongoing support these patients require. Valuable time was then released for the doctors to devote to diagnosis, decisions regarding treatment and research.

Day et al. (1970)) and Lewis and Resmick (1967) found that, where patients had been cared for by both physician and nurse practitioner, they seemed to prefer to go on seeing the nurse. Hill et al. (1991) confirms that the nurse practitioner is an effective practitioner who is acceptable to patients and a valuable member of the outpatient team.

In four of the hospitals visited the role of the nurse practitioner was established and accepted.

Research

The 1989 *Strategy for Nursing* advocates that nurses foster a receptive attitude to research and be committed to pursuing and applying it in the delivery of health care. Moreover, DOH *Research for Health* papers (1991, 1993b) emphasize the use of research findings in health care. *Vision for the Future* (1993a) stresses that credibility of future care will depend on a number of factors including sound research.

Nurses would not dispute the value of research and yet few are fully conversant with all the latest projects applicable to their own speciality. Even fewer actually take part in research. The metrologists in the hospitals in this survey were mostly involved in collecting data for drug trials and medical research. The information regarding any research findings was rarely given to other nurses. In fact, there were complaints regarding the lack of communication between the metrologists and the rest of the nursing staff.

In one hospital, the metrologist's role had developed in response to patient needs and had eventually evolved into that of nurse practitioner. Research which also concerned the development of nursing practice became an integral part of their work.

One hospital in Sweden had set up a very well staffed and equipped research centre for nurses where they could receive help with small projects and those leading to higher academic qualifications.

Four hospitals were actively engaged in nursing research.

Conclusion

In the hospitals included in this project the services and quality of care for rheumatic patients varied considerably from region to region. Some had much better facilities than others, and the number of consultant posts per head of population varied from region to region and between the two countries, Sweden being by far the better served in terms of specialists available.

The role of the nurse at every level varied from the 'laissez-faire' style of management observed in some outpatient clinics, to those who acted as change agents, innovators and skilled professional nurses. Some of the criteria used to assess the quality of care given to patients involved all members of the multidisciplinary team. Others showed how nurses can play an active team role and introduce good practices of their own. They had taken on the role described by Pigg (1985) of primary responsibility for the comprehensive management of each patient.

Survey of these ten hospitals gave the following outcomes (Fig 4.6):

- The quality of patient care bore no relationship to the size of population, or to the number of consultants in each district.
- The number of specialist nurses from sister upwards did not affect the quality of care given by themselves or the junior nursing staff.
- Five hospitals demonstrated their commitment to the criteria chosen to assess the units. In four hospitals, nurses at specialist, practitioner or consultant level were in post. In one hospital in Sweden, although this post did not exist, the head nurse in charge of the outpatient clinic was chairman of the Swedish Rheumatology Association and had, entirely through her own efforts and against great opposition, instigated every single one of the practices listed for that hospital, in her own department.

The final conclusion drawn from information accumulated and analysed, was that if a role equivalent to that of nurse specialist was in post, the staff in that unit were more innovative and forward thinking. The specialist nurse was a prime motivator for improving the quality of care for patients with rheumatic diseases.

The role of the rheumatology nurse practitioner

A report which included a description of the hospitals visited, a resumé and critique of its findings and a summary of the suggested role for a rheumatology

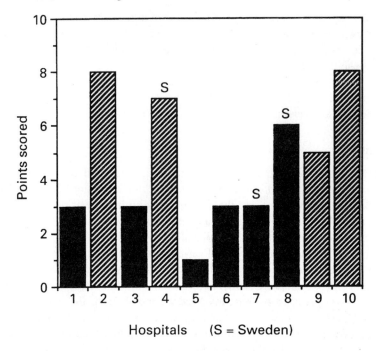

Figure 4.6   Evaluation criteria showing the influence of the nurse practitioner/specialist ▨ Nurse – Consultant Practitioner Specialist; ■ Senior nurse 'specialist' not in post.

nurse practitioner within the organization, was submitted at the end of a period of 4 months' sabbatical leave. Nurse management accepted the recommendations in the report and, acknowledging the deficiencies in the nursing care of rheumatic patients, appointed the first rheumatology nurse practitioner in the hospital. Consultant medical staff were not united in their support of this new role, but it was possible, with the encouragement of one consultant and the nursing staff, to improve quality of care for the patients during the first year of the appointment.

Defining the role

The titles of 'practitioner' and 'specialist' are used here interchangeably, although it is accepted that there is a need for these designations to be clarified and defined. Several roles are now universally accepted as being appropriate for the nurse practititioner.

Practitioner/direct care provider

Maycock (1990) feels that to have any credibility the specialist must have a case load of his or her own and thus be seen to act as patient advocate and role model. Calkin (1984) describes an expert nurse as being able to assess and intervene in varied client responses.

Educator

Dirschel (1976) and Metcalf et al. (1984) describe a staff educator role. Blount et al. (1981) suggest that they may use their teaching skills by assisting in the development of patient education materials. Fife and Lemner (1983) propose that they should alert other members of the multidisciplinary team to nursing's unique role in meeting patients' needs.

Consultant

As early as 1977, Blake was referring to a clinical nurse specialist who might function as an expert consultant or process consultant (Blake, 1977). Maycock (1990) indicates a nurse able to act as a point of referral for other professionals as well as for the patients and families.

Researcher

The *Strategy for Nursing* (1989c) advocated the need for research to underpin and make the innovations in nursing tenable. Fife and Lemler (1983) are in agreement that, at the most basic level, the nurse specialist should be able to interpret research findings and make use of research to improve practice. The next step would be to act as research collaborator and co-ordinator.

Change agent

The role of change agent is very often the most difficult to fulfil, particularly as the practitioner is very often in an independent role outside the accepted line positions of the organization. Everson (1981) expected the role to be that of a catalyst and Gordon (1969) saw them promoting professional growth and independence rather than simple compliance and identification. Gordon (1969) also recognized the difficulties of bringing about change without the support of peers and administrators.

Putting theory into practice

Deciding on a set of criteria by which to assess rheumatology units and the role of a specialist nurse who could have a major role in introducing these criteria, is comparatively easy. State of the art information is more prolific than in the past when rheumatology nursing as a speciality was in its infancy. The RCN Rheumatology Forum and The British Health Professionals in Rheumatology (BHPR) offer not only the means of acquiring up-to-date information on the subject, but through their conferences and study days provide opportunities for nurses to meet and exchange ideas. Much time at these meetings is spent on debating how to bring about change and introduce modern, well researched practices. Discussions with other rheumatology nurses reveal that, in their role as change agents many, as Everson (1981) suggests, have experienced opposition and have been forced to rethink and adapt in order to get the best possible deal for the patient.

The opportunity to develop the practitioner role grew primarily from the recognition of patient needs in a busy drug monitoring clinic. The original criteria and the perceived role of specialist nurse, although adapted and reshaped as events unfolded, provided useful guidelines and remained the essence of the eventual outcomes.

Analysing a drug monitoring clinic

The guidelines which had been developed formed a useful base from which to reshape the role of the nurse practitioner to meet patients' needs. The clinic in question had routinely 40–50 patients attending each Monday morning who were seen by one consultant rheumatologist and one senior house officer. During 1 month, for four consecutive Mondays, several aspects of the clinic were examined and summarized.

a) Pattern of attendance at the clinics to include:
   - number of patients attending clinic
   - number of patients not attending (DNA)
   - number of new patients (NP)
   - number of patients on disease modifying anti-rheumatic drugs (DMARDS) requiring monitoring (DRUG MON)
   - number of patients on DMARDS with problems requiring a medical opinion (PROBLEMS)
   - number of patients not on DMARDS but requiring clinic appointments (OTHER)

b) The frequency of appointments:
   - 6-weekly   (6/52)
   - 1 month   (1/12)
   - 2-monthly   (2/12)
   - 3-monthly   (3/12)
   - 6-monthly   (6/12)

c) Summary of the DMARDS prescribed:
   - methotrexate   (MTX)
   - penicillamine   (D. PEN)
   - myocrisin   (GOLD)
   - sulphasalazine   (SASP)
   - azathioprine   (AZA)

Figure 4.7 illustrates the pattern of attendance at one of the Monday clinic sessions. With slight variations a similar trend was repeated in the other three sessions.

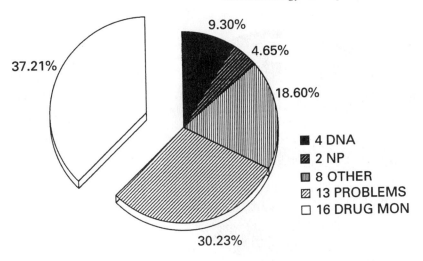

Figure 4.7 Pattern of attendance observed in a drug monitoring clinic

Looking at the frequency of appointments and list of DMARDS prescribed for the 16 patients (37.21%) who had come to clinic to have their blood results monitored, produced the information demonstrated in Figs 4.8 and 4.9.

Examining the attendance of those 16 patients revealed that, although appointments varied slightly from time to time, they did attend with approximately the same regularity over the space of a year. In this particular sample, one patient came 6-weekly, four at 2-monthly, four at 3-monthly and six at monthly intervals.

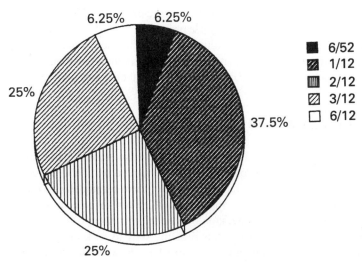

Figure 4.8 Frequency of appointments

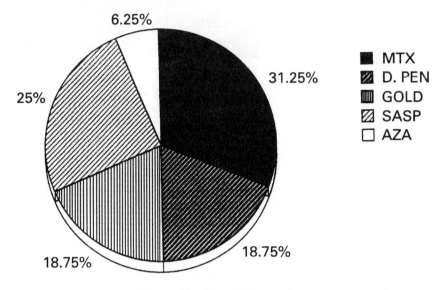

Figure 4.9 DMARDS prescribed

The other patient came once a year and was monitored by the general practitioner throughout the rest of the year (Fig. 4.8).

Evaluation of the different types of DMARDS taken by this group of patients revealed that the five major drugs in this category were prescribed by the consultant, although some more often than others, in particular, methotrexate was used the most. In the session chosen, five patients were taking methotrexate, three penicillamine, three myocrisin, four sulphasalazine and one azathioprine.

After this preliminary examination of the organization of the clinic the conclusion arrived at by the consultant and the nurse practitioner was that approximately 30% of patients came to clinic for drug monitoring only, that these patients were comparatively well and that there was no reason why they could not be monitored in general practice. Guidelines initiating GP monitoring were then drawn up (Fig. 4.10).

Drug protocols

It is generally recognized that the easiest way to ensure that patients are monitored efficiently is to formulate protocols which are agreed upon and understood by all members of staff who would have need to use them as guidelines. Protocols cannot be fully comprehensive in that they will never be able to anticipate every eventuality. Nevertheless, they should be extensive enough to ensure maximum patient safety and they should encourage the staff to seek help if there is doubt regarding continuation of treatment. Figure 4.11 shows a sample of a protocol for methotrexate.

1	Patients should have been taking the drug for at least **3 months**.
2	During this time the patient would have seen the Rheumatology Consultant and the Rheumatology Nurse at least once.
3	Blood and urine tests should be within normal limits.
4	Patients would have received the relevant information and education regarding their condition and the drugs prescribed for them and would understand the importance of complying with the requirements of monitoring.
5	The patient would be given a diary to record drug dosage and blood results. They would be given contact phone numbers and encouraged to ring the nurse practitioner for support and help.
6	The consultant would send a letter and appropriate protocol to the GP requesting they take over the drug monitoring for the patient.
7	The nurse practitioner would send a letter and protocol to the practice nurse requesting help in monitoring the patient.

Figure 4.10   Criteria for commencing GP monitoring of patients on DMARDS

Up until this stage in the reorganization of the clinic, ideas had flowed, enthusiasm abounded and the future outlook appeared optimistic. However, two obstacles emerged and threatened to frustrate further progress – the reluctance of the patients to relinquish medical, hospital based monitoring, and lack of information regarding the knowledge and confidence of the practice nurses. Both these problems were therefore addressed.

Patient education and empowerment

After the decision had been made to encourage a 'shared care' approach to drug monitoring, the task of identifying those patients who had been stabilized and were well enough to be monitored in the community was assigned to the nurse practitioner. The final decision regarding choice of patient remained with the consultant, but because of the original agreed criteria, a mutual understanding very quickly developed between the consultant and practitioner and there was seldom disagreement concerning selection.

Introducing the patients to the idea of shared monitoring was done in stages. Initially, the consultant selected patients he or she wished to return to the community and these began to see the nurse practitioner at each visit. Not all patients welcomed this change. Some felt that they were being deprived of expert care. The development of relationships between patient and nurse at this point became crucial to the success of the new system.

Methotrexate

Dose range: 2.5–25 mg per week

Administration: Oral or intramuscular

Monitoring:	**Initially:**	Fortnightly FBC & ESR Monthly U&Es & LFTs
	After 3 months:	Monthly FBC, ESR, U&Es, LFTs

Please record results in patient's monitoring booklet

Potential side effects:	**Management:**
Nausea	Add anti-emetic. Consider reduction in MTX dose
Reduced WBC <3.0 × 10/1	Stop MTX Contact RNP
Reduced platelet count <140 × 10/1	Stop MTX Contact RNP
Reduced Hb <8 g/dl	Contact RNP
Increased MCV	Check folate
Increased LFTs – AST > 120	Stop MTX Contact RNP
Raised serum creatinine >115 mmol/l	Stop MTX Contact RNP
Mouth ulcers	If severe stop MTX Difflam mouth wash Check folate Folinic acid 15 mg qds 48 h

Rheumatology Nurse Practitioner

....(Name, telephone, bleep number)

Consultant Rheumatologist

....(Name and telephone number)

Figure 4.11   Drug monitoring in patients with rheumatoid arthritis

The first appointment to see the nurse practitioner could sometimes last from 15 to 20 minutes, whilst the patient's knowledge base of their disease and coping strategies were determined. Information and education in the form of verbal and written material were offered at this stage. Usually, information was in the form of Arthritis and Rheumatism Council (ARC) and Arthritis Care (AC) leaflets, but any other problems were addressed and, if necessary, each patient was contacted by phone or letter to resolve any outstanding questions.

At the second appointment, the patient was given an information leaflet and record diary, specific to the drug they were taking. The entries in the diary were explained and the importance of drug monitoring compliance emphasized. They were given a phone and bleep number for the nurse practitioner and encouraged to make contact whenever the need arose.

By the third visit, in most instances, patients had confidence in the nurse practitioner's knowledge and ability to cope with their ongoing care. Some began to state a preference to see the nurse. They expressed appreciation of the time spent in answering their questions. Such statements as 'no-one ever explained these things to me before, now I understand', 'I found the information you gave very useful', 'I feel I am in control now', or 'I am able to explain my disease to my relatives'. Female patients said they found the discussion of sexual problems with a female nurse less embarrassing.

Most patients were coming to the monitoring clinic at monthly or 6-weekly intervals. (Fig 4.8). By the end of the first 3 months, the nurse–patient relationship had evolved to the extent that it was possible to discuss the induction of GP monitoring with a number of patients. Each patient was given a pro-forma letter with the appropriate protocol to be taken to the practice nurse before the end of the next 4 weeks. At the same time, the consultant sent a pro-forma letter and protocol to the GP asking for help in monitoring the patient. Both letters emphasized the need to contact the hospital if the practice had any difficulty in complying with the terms of the protocol. The patient was also encouraged to contact the nurse practitioner for help and support.

After the first 6 months, 53 patients had been sent for monitoring to 31 GP practices. Only two practices refused to do the monitoring. On average, these patients were attending the clinic and being seen by the doctor at 6-weekly intervals. By sharing the care with GPs attendances for these patients, alone was reduced by 318 follow-up appointments in 1 year. In less than 1 year the consultant was able to reduce clinic follow-up appointments from 35 to 25 in each session and increase new patient appointments from 2 to 3 each session and at the same time be able to accommodate demands for urgent new and follow-up appointments.

Practice nurse development

As the roles of purchaser and provider become evident, the division which existed between community and hospital is no longer tenable. Moreover, if patients are to receive the expert attention and care to which they are entitled, and which is now mandatory vis-a-vis the Patients' Charter, communication and co-operation is essential.

Practice nurses are expected to be experts in a number of fields. Communication of information from GP to practice nurse cannot always be guaranteed. It is up to the nurses who are specialists in each discipline to make sure that they are vigilant in passing on information to their colleagues in the community.

Initial contact with the local university generated instant rewards. The offer of a session on rheumatic conditions to include information on drugs and drug monitoring was immediately taken up. Feedback from the first group of 30 practice nurses was that the session was interesting, practical and contained useful information relevant to their area of practice. The session is now included in every practice nurse course.

A questionnaire was then designed to ascertain the needs of practice nurses (Fig. 4.12). The 31 practices involved in drug monitoring at the time and all other practices who shared the care of patients with the consultant were targeted. It was obvious, after the first few questionnaires were returned, that there was a need for more knowledge concerning rheumatology. Most were in favour of a study day: some requested a one-to-one session with the practitioner, a few favoured small group learning situations.

A little over 6 months after the first patients went out to the community, the first full day study day was organized for practice nurses at the local university. It included an overview and update of the speciality of rheumatology and of drugs in common usage to treat the diseases, a look at the problems encountered in general practice, sessions from nurse practitioners regarding aspects of their work, as well as the work of ARC and last, but not least, the views of a patient (Fig. 4.12).

Planning for the future – continuing the journey

> There is a certain relief in change, even though it be from bad to worse; as I have found in travelling in a stage-coach, that it is often a comfort to shift one's position and be bruised in a new place
>
> Washington Irving, (1783–1859) *Tales of a traveller*: Preface.

The reasons for starting this journey were put before you at the beginning of this chapter. Many of the details concerning difficulties encountered during the development of the role have been omitted. This was partly because such details would have filled the book, but mostly because the aim of the chapter was to show that there is always a way forward, despite the opposition and difficulty encountered by nurses when trying to develop these roles.

Irving's (1969) experiences readily relate to the ordeals of the chronic arthritis sufferer, but they can also be applied to the nurse who takes up their cause and specializes in arthritic conditions. It is neither a glamorous nor an emotional cause to champion. Often ideas have to be abandoned and other routes taken because of lack of support. This can be painful and soul destroying and requires a formidable determination to go on. Sometimes, as suggested by Bond (1993), it is easier to bring about change in smaller establishments – like Burford in Oxford (Pearson, 1988), than to take on the complex, hierarchical, traditional social systems of the

QUESTIONNAIRE FOR PRACTICE NURSES

We are trying to improve the ways in which you receive information regarding the care of rheumatology patients. Could you please help us to evaluate our service to you by answering the following questions.

PLEASE PUT APPROPRIATE LETTER IN BOXES UNLESS ASKED OTHERWISE

1) Were you aware of the existence of a Rheumatology Nurse Practitioner at the Hospital?
  (a) yes
  (b) no

2) If yes to question 1, how did you receive this information?
....
....

3) Do you find it easy to contact the Rheumatology Nurse Practitioner?
  a) yes   b) requires more than one phone call
  c) no   d) not applicable

4) What kind of service do you require from the nurse practitioner?
  a) advisory   b) educational   (tick those applicable)
  d) home visits   c) supportive

5) How would you prefer to liaise with the nurse practitioner?
                                              (tick those applicable)
  a) by phone
  b) by letter
  c) visit the hospital yourself
  d) expect the nurse practitioner to visit you

6) Would you like further information to be given to you? (tick those applicable)
  a) on a one to one basis
  b) in small groups/short session
  c) in the form of study days

7) Would you find it beneficial to receive more information regarding the care of patients with rheumatoid disease?
  a) yes
  b) no

8) If the answer to question **7** is yes, how would you prefer this information to be given?   (tick those applicable)
  a) on a one to one basis
  b) in small groups, short sessions
  c) in the form of study days

FOR FUTURE COMMUNICATION PLEASE SUPPLY:
FULL NAME .... ·
PRACTICE ADDRESS..
....
....
....

THANK YOU FOR TAKING THE TIME TO ANSWER THIS QUESTIONNAIRE ·

RHEUMATOLOGY NURSE PRACTITIONER
TEL. NO.............................
DIRECT LINE...................
BLEEP...............................

© S.M.O'GORMAN MAY 1993

Figure 4.12 Questionnaire for practice nurses

large teaching hospitals. Those who become truly involved in this speciality, support and work alongside their clients. The pity of it is, the patients themselves are very much aware of their low status in today's brave new world.

The Patients' Charter – the way forward

The Patients' Charter sets out rights and standards which set out the principles for the future development of the NHS. In a speciality such as rheumatology it presents nurses with the opportunity to improve delivery of care. The charter talks of a service that

- 'always puts the patient first . . . in ways responsive to people's views and needs;
- provides services that produce clear, measurable benefits to people's health, with more emphasis than in the past on health promotion and prevention;
- is highly efficient, representing really good value for money;
- respects and values the immense resource of skill and dedication which is to be found amongst those who work for and with the National Health Service' (DOH, 1991b).

The reorganization of the drug monitoring clinic reflects the themes of the Patients' Charter. From the start, the patient's needs were paramount and when shared care was introduced, it was tailored to suit individual requirements. In many instances patients were given knowledge and information that had not been available to them before. They were encouraged to question treatment, develop self help strategies, become health rather than illness orientated and enhance their own control of the disease.

Those patients who were on 6-monthly appointments, now see the nurse practitioner once a year and the consultant once a year. Assessment of the patient includes a Health Assessment Questionnaire (HAQ) grip strength, pain and early morning stiffness scores are used by the nurse to evaluate progress. The appointment also provides further opportunity for communication and support.

That the organization of shared care provides an efficient, value for money service is self evident. Patients now have a team involving hospital and community staff, communicating well, sharing knowledge and between them providing improved quality care. A great deal of the liaison between team members falls to the nurse practitioner and the difference this post can make is represented by Maycock (1990) in Fig. 4.13. Patients who hitherto gave time, energy and money to constant trips to hospital, sometimes spending most of a day in pain and discomfort in an ambulance, can, if they wish, visit their own GP or have their blood taken by the district nurse if they are housebound.

Acknowledging the skill and dedication of staff in the community was of paramount importance to the success of this scheme. Letters sent out to the GP and practice nurse were carefully worded, help and assistance offered rather than imposed. The questionnaire brought further information regarding education and updating requirements of the practice nurses.

Could any of this have been introduced long before? Reorganizing a busy outpatient clinic is rather like trying to service a car engine when it is being driven at 70 miles an hour down the motorway. Trying to spot the problems and come up with answers, when large numbers of patients are coming to clinic and have to be seen, advised or treated by the staff, leaves little time for major reorganizations.

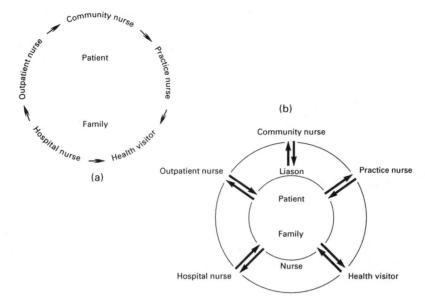

Figure 4.13   (a) The bewildering variety of nurses; (b) the introduction of rheumatology nurse specialists and its effects, from Maycock (1990)

Because of a mutual respect for each other's knowledge and skills, the consultant and nurse practitioner were able to work together in this instance and facilitate the changes. Support, knowledge, opportunity and determination, elements necessary for the realization of change, could then be put in place enabling the nurse practitioner to became the catalyst for the transformation.

Unexpected dividends

One of the most rewarding innovations of the first year came out of the formation of a support group in the community. As professionals, it is easy to lose sight of what are the real needs of our patients. Education programmes are difficult to set up in the hospital. Inpatient periods longer than 2 weeks are becoming increasingly rare. Patients are not always at their receptive best whilst in hospital. It is often when they return home that they need most support and would benefit from further information. Most people with arthritis never occupy a hospital bed. Some do not ever see a rheumatology specialist. Moreover, people with arthritis will tell you that the most useful conversations are those they have with fellow sufferers – only they have the experience to be able to assure each other.

It was with these thoughts in mind that a branch of ARC was formed. Facilitated by the nurse practitioner initially, it is now organized, run by and for people with arthritis, their friends and relatives. The monthly meetings combine social with information events; at the same time money is raised for ARC.

Another innovation developed from the realization that from the original list of criteria used to assess the units visited, staff education and update had been omitted. The enthusiastic practitioner can overlook the fact that most of the staff dealing with these patients in hospital or community will not have had any formal training in rheumatology. Study days and the input into practice nurse courses can certainly help, but a speciality as wide as this, affecting so many of the population, should surely have a higher profile in the initial training of nurses.

It has therefore been decided that a rheumatology module will be developed at a local education establishment with the nurse practitioner as course leader and adviser.

Conclusion

Hopefully, this chapter will encourage others to join the ranks of the rheumatology nurse practitioner. Perhaps the most important fact to remember is that, as a disease, arthritis rarely kills. An American sufferer was quoted by the National Commission in 1978 as saying, 'The most profound thing anyone ever told me about rheumatoid arthritis is that it wouldn't kill me, but it sure would make me wish I was dead ... '. During the lifetime of a patient there is much for the nurse to do and much to learn.

> Today is not yesterday; we ourselves change; how can our Works and Thoughts, if they are always to be the fittest, continue always the same? Change, indeed is painful; yet ever needful; and if memory have its force and worth, so also has Hope.
>
> Carlyle (1795–1881) *Essays: Characteristics*

Useful addresses

Arthritis and Rheumatism
Council for Research
Head Office
Copeman Street
St. Mary's Court
St. Mary's Gate
Chesterfield
Derbyshire, S41 7TD

Arthritis Care
18 Stephenson Way
London, NW1 2HD

RCN Rheumatology Nurses' Forum
RCN Advisor in Rheumatology Nursing,
RCN Headquarters,
20 Cavendish Square,
London, W1M 0AB.

British Health Professionals
   in Rheumatology, (BHPR)
3 St. Andrews Place,
Regents Park,
London, NW1 4LB.

References

Altoff B, Nordenskiold U (1985) *Joint Protection*. Pharmacia, Sweden.
Bird HA, le Gallez P, Hill J (1985) *Combined Care of the Rheumatic Patient*. Heidelberg: Springer.

Blake P (1977) The clinical nurse specialist as nurse consultant. *Journal of Nursing Administration*; **7(10)**: 33–36.

Blount M, Burge S, Crigler L, Finklemeir B, Sanborn C (1981) Extending the influence of clinical nurse specialist. *Nursing Administration Quarterly*; **6910**: 53–63.

Bolt D (1983) Why we are worried about the process. *Nursing Times*; **Aug. 24**: 11–12.

Bond S (1993) Extending the range of primary nursing. *Nursing Standard*; **7** [46]: 25–28.

Bowling A (1991) *Measuring Health*. Milton Keynes: Open University Press.

Calkin J (1984) A model for advanced nursing practice. *Journal of Advanced Nursing Administration*, **14** [1]: 24–30.

Carlyle T (1869) *Critical and Miscellaneous Essays: Collected and Republished by Carlyle, T*. London: Chapman & Hall.

Chesson S (1984) Social and emotional aspects of rheumatoid arthritis. *Nursing* (Oxford); **2**: 914–917.

Day LR, Engli R, Silver HK (1970) Acceptance of pediatric nurse practitioners: parents' opinion of combined care by a pediatrician and pediatric nurse practitioner in private practice. *Amercian Journal of diseases of Children* **119**: 204–208.

DHSS (1990) *Hospital Year Book*. London: HMSO.

Dirschel KM (1976) The conception, gestation and delivery of the clinical nurse specialist. In:*Quality Patient Care and the Role of the Clinical Nurse Specialist*. New York: Wiley.

DOH (1989a) *Working for Patients*. London: HMSO.

DOH (1989b) *Caring for People*. London: HMSO.

DOH (1989c) *A Strategy for Nursing*. London: HMSO.

DOH (1990) *NHS Management Executive. The role of nurses and other non-medical staff in outpatient departments*. Middlesex: DOH Publications.

DOH (1991a) *Research for Health*. London: HMSO.

DOH (1991b) *The Patients' Charter*. London: HMSO.

DOH (1993a) *Vision for the Future*. London: HMSO.

DOH (1993b) *Research for Health*. London: HMSO.

Everson S (1981) Integration of the role of clinical nurse specialist. *Journal of Continuing Education in Nursing*, **12** [2]: 16–19.

Farmer E (1986) Exploring the issues, In: Kershaw B, Salvage J (eds) *Models for Nursing*. New York: Wiley.

Fenton M (1985) Identifying competencies of clinical nurse specialists. *Journal of Nursing Administration*; **15** [12]: 31–37.

Fife B, Lemler S (1983) The psychiatric nurse specialist: a valuable asset in a general hospital. *Journal of Nursing Administration*; **13** [4]: 14–17.

Gordon M (1969) The clinical nurse specialist as change agent. *Nursing Outlook*; **17** [3]: 37–39.

Gutch R, Cope D (1992) *Countdown to Community Care*. London: Arthritis Care.

Hegyvary ST (1982) *The Change to Primary Nursing*. St Louis: Mosby.

Hill J (1985) Nursing clinics for arthritis. *Nursing Times*; **81**: 33–34.

Hill J (1986) Patient evaluation of a rheumatology nursing clinic. *Nursing Times*; **82**: 42–43.

Hill J, Bird HA, Harmer R, Wright V (1991) A comparative study of a traditional medical and nurse practitioner clinic. *British Journal of Rheumatology*; **xxx** suppl. 1, April, 2.

HMSO (1991) National Audit Office, NHS Outpatient Services, HC 191, London.

HMSO (1992) *The Health of the Nation*. London: HMSO.

Irving W (1969) Tales of a traveler (1824). In: Pochmann HA (ed.), *The Complete Works of Washington Irving*. Wisconsin: University of Wisconsin Press.

Jette AM (1982) Improving patient co-operation with arthritis treatment regimens. *Arthritis and Rheumatism*; **25**: 447–453.

Johnson S (1775) The laws of ecclesiastical polity, quoting Hooker R. in preface to *Dictionary of the English Language*.

Kirwan RJ, Reeback JS (1983) Using a modified Stanford Health Assessment

Questionnaire to assess disability in UK patients with rheumatoid arthritis. *Annals of Rheumatic Diseases*; **42**: 219–220.

le Gallez P (1984) Patient education and self management. *Nursing* (Oxford); **2**: 916–917.

Lewis CE, Resmick BA (1967) Nurse clinics and progressive ambulatory care. *New England Journal of Medicine*; **277**: 1236–1241.

Lo Bindo-Wood G, Haber J (1986) *Nursing Research: Critical Appraisal and Utilisation.* St. Louis: CV Mosby.

Lorig K, Fries JF (1993) *The Arthritis Helpbook – what you can do for your arthritis.* London: Souvenir Press.

MacDonald ET, MacDonald JB (1982) *Drug Treatment in the Elderly.* Chichester: Wiley.

Macfarlane A (1985) When givers prove unkind. *Nursing Mirror*, **161**, [14]: 36–37.

Manthey M, Ciske K, Robertson P, Harris R (1970) Primary Nurse: a return to the concept of 'my nurse' and 'my patient'. *Nursing Forum*; **9** [1]: 65–83.

Marsden E (1992) Outpatient nurses must adapt to survive. *British Journal of Nursing*; **1** [7]: 356–357.

Maycock J (1990) A catalyst for better rheumatology care. *Nursing Standard*; **4** [50]: 54–55.

Metcalf J, Werner M, Richmond T (1984) The clinical nurse specialist in the clinical career ladder. *Nursing Administration Quarterly*; **9** [1]: 9–19.

Morris K, Schweiger J (1979) Clinical nurse specialist role creation: an acheivable goal. *Nursing Administration Quarterly*; **4** [1]: 67–78.

Neuberger GB (1984) The role of the nurse with arthritis patients on drug therapy. *Nursing Clinics of North America* (Philadelphia); **19**: 593–604.

Oldham J, Tallis R, Howe T, Smith G, Petterson T (1992) Objective assessment of muscle function. *Nursing Standard*; **6** [45]: 37–39

Pagana KD, Pagana TJ (eds) (1982) *Diagnostic Testing and Nursing Implication, a Case Study Approach.* St Louis: CV Mosby.

Pearson A (1988) *Primary Nursing: Nursing in the Burfoot and Oxford Nursing Development Units.* London: Croom Helm.

Pigg JS (1989) Role of nursing and allied professionals in the treatment of arthritis. In: McCarty DJ (ed), *Arthritis and Allied Conditions: a Textbook of Rheumatology*, 11th edn. Philadelphia: Lea & Fibiger.

Pigg JS (1990) Rheumatology nursing: evolution of the role and function of a subspeciality. *Arthritis Care and Research*; **3** [3]: 109–115.

Pigg JS, Driscoll PW, Caniff R (1985) *Rheumatology Nursing – a Problem Orientated Approach.* Chichester: Wiley Medical.

Powe A (1993) Nursing theory vs nursing practice. *Senior Nurse*; **13** [5]: 32–34.

Rafferty AM (1986) Teamwork or threat. *Senior Nurse*; **4** [1]: 22–23.

Ritchie DM, Boyle JA, McInnes JM, Jasani MK, Dalakos TG, Grieveson P, Buchanan WW (1968) Clinical studies with an articular index for the assessmetnt of joint tenderness in patients with rheumatoid arthritis. *Quarterly Journal of Medicine*; **37**: 393–406.

Salvage J (1985) *Politics of Nursing.* London: Heinemann.

Schober J 1993 Frameworks for nursing practice. In: Hinchcliffe SM, Norman SE, Schober JE (eds), *Nursing Practice and Health Care.* London: Edward Arnold.

UKCC 1993 *The Council's Proposed Standards for Post-Registration Education.* Annexe Two to Registrar's Letter 8/1993: 5–6.

Wood P (1986) *Arthritis and Rheumatism in the Eighties.* Chesterfield: Arthritis and Rheumatism Council.

Wright V (1982) Multi-purpose therapist or multi-professional teams. *Occupational Therapist*; **45**: 229–230.

Section II

Models and Frameworks for Developing Practice

Practitioners have always placed great emphasis upon achieving excellence in the delivery of care. This has created an image of isolated individuals 'beavering' away without ever sharing the benefits of innovation with colleagues in other areas. Some nurses may publish their ideas in professional journals or speak at conferences. The frenetic existence of professional life, however, means that many practitioners just do not have the time to devote to such pursuits. In Chapter 5, Weir and Kendrick confront this problem and describe the pragmatics involved in developing a network specifically designed as a forum where people may meet to talk about practice. The remit of the network, however, is much broader than the value of meeting and talking. What has evolved from these meetings is a dynamic series of themes and events which not only means the sharing of innovative practice but the setting of a challenging agenda for future developments. The central thrust of the chapter is to give other nurses a framework for developing networks in their own area.

A key element in accountable and responsible practice is the ability to demonstrate current, ongoing and reflective practice which is founded upon a strong research base. In Chapter 6, Rosser confronts the negative themes which are often presented by the theory–practice gap and discusses a method of learning which is directly linked to the pragmatic realities of care delivery. What emerges from this is a dynamic chapter which presents the theoretical and practical considerations involved in a challenging approach to learning.

The last 10 years has seen a radical shift in the political themes underpinning the National Health Service. This has led to the position where health care delivery is now governed by the influence of market forces. The emergence of a market-based model has created a culture which is geared towards a cost-effective equation. In Chapter 7, Hale and Hampson grapple with the challenges involved in reconciling a budget-focused service with total quality management. What emerges from this is a stimulating discussion which describes a framework for achieving total quality management within a business-centred environment.

In the final chapter in this section, Shea and Leather discuss the theoretical challenges which have accompanied a renaissance in the popularity of complementary therapies. Using an analytical and reflective approach, the authors examine the role of medicine as the dominant means of delivering health care. What emerges from this is a picture of health care that portrays orthodox medicine as a powerful protagonist to which all other approaches to health must play an acquiescent role. Such themes are challenged by Shea and Leather, who argue that complementary therapies can play an essential part in acting as a conduit for increasing the therapeutic options available to patients. Emerging from this is an argument for nurses to play a vital role in bringing the therapeutic value of complementary therapies to the forefront of care giving.

The common theme throughout this section is one of innovative thinking. If practice is to be dynamic, then it must be preceded by cogent ideas which are tempered with pragmatic realism. What emerges from this is a collection of thoughts which have influenced nurses to think about the frameworks and models which help form and influence their work.

The Editors
1994

5 Networking: method, model and application

Pauline Weir and Kevin Kendrick

Because a whole is more powerful than the sum of its parts, the dynamics of the developing network are more effective than the individual members alone. The collaborative process seems to provide an abundance of creative energy for implementing change. Ideas and strategies literally bounce off each other as the network serves as a resource for growth and progress.

(Carr, 1982)

Innovation and change are high on the nursing profession's agenda. This is reflected in the abundance of new themes surrounding clinical, educational and managerial practice. A central aspect in all these areas of development is the emerging role of the nurse as a change agent (Wright, 1990).

The focus and direction of this chapter is to discuss the evolution and implementation of a network for facilitating excellence and change in the different spheres of nursing. This process will begin with an exploration of those theoretical, political and contemporary events which provided the impetus for this endeavour.

Beginnings

The process of networking can be defined within the *Concise Oxford English Dictionary* (1990) 'as a group of people who exchange information, contacts and experience for professional or social purposes'.

Historically, Umiker (1989) reminds us the term used to refer to men who had 'connections in the office' or 'on the golf course'. He also cites the well known phrase 'it's not what you know, but who you know that counts'. However, a more contemporary view by Murphy (1988) says 'it's not what you know, but who you know and who knows you that really counts!'.

The art of networking involves creating relationships and applies to both men and women in differing spheres (Umiker, 1989). Many authors agree that people who value networking share common goals and interests (Ferguson, 1980; McKendrick, 1982; Anderson et al., 1983; Wake and Vogel, 1985; Smith, 1987; Murphy, 1988; Harter et al., 1989; Fain and Viau, 1989; Hockenberry-Eaton, 1992).

These themes are expanded by Hunt et al. (1983), who describe networking as a 'high level group process, a creative thinking group'. According to McCray (1986), networking is a prerequisite for transforming beliefs and values into 'attainable goals'. This view is supported by Harter et al. (1989), who refers to the usefulness of networks going beyond the stage of information exchanges to result in aspects of change within a system.

The idea of people coming together to discuss and debate mutual interests is not alien to nursing. As O'Connor (1982) states, 'many advances for the profession are the result of a core of nurses working together to identify and use resources to solve problems and promote ideas'. She continues by saying 'networking is a new term for the old process of using your contacts and knowing who to know'.

The connotations of networking have their origins in organizational theory. Reflecting the essence and direction of this term, Lynch (1993) states 'The process is self generating and self-organizing. It consists of people communicating, sharing ideas and information, and offering support and direction to each other. This leads to the establishment of specific networks that can foster the building of a positive power base. Networks work with other networks and thus have tremendous power for directing change'. The essence of these terms is reflected in a plethora of seminal and contemporary literature which explores how the networking process can be achieved.

Who are the networkers?

Networking is no longer solely within the male domain, as both men and women in any profession can access a networking system. 'Networking is an essential mechanism for personal, professional and practice development' (Mackereth et al., 1994). They add 'it can happen through professional courses, local forums, courses, conferences and so on'.

According to Meisenhelder (1982), networking is needed to function at three levels within nursing. She highlights 'networking at grass roots level is most crucial to the unity and survival of the profession'. This is best conducted at first level registration to support colleagues and influence practice. A second level of networking is required amongst nurses at leadership level. Sharing and supporting one another at this level reinforces a positive environment which staff are motivated to work in. Finally, a third political level is referred by which nurses can utilize the networking process. Imagine the largest section of the NHS workforce actively striving for a similar change at a political level, as Meisenhelder says 'their impact would be colossal'.

Every nurse can value the process of networking; no one is excluded. Within the different levels McCray (1986) emphasizes 'a positive attitude about networking and sharing reflects a personal and professional pride'. Nurses are not confined to only one network, but membership of different groups can enhance the networking process.

Developing networks

Networks are created to fulfil a need. In the words of Lynch (1993), 'It is during times of intense change, when individuals and groups have feelings of insecurity, powerlessness, and loss of control, that networks begin to emerge. Networks represent linkages between and among those who recognize mutual threats, problems, needs and goals that cannot be resolved or satisfied by traditional structures and relationships'. Successful networks cannot develop without a purpose and a great deal of planning. According to Kitson (1993), networks develop when the following factors occur simultaneously:

- a topic of mutual interest occupies the intellect and imagination of a significant number of people;
- debates and deliberations indicate a set of shared values or a working philosophy on a topic;
- a leader or leaders emerge who is/are prepared to organize the previously informal group of like-minded interested people.

Drawing upon these themes, Hunt et al. (1983) describe five developmental stages in the formation of a network:

1 idea initiation
    - The idea initiator may gather a group of people together with 'a notion that a group approach or network of experts can accomplish a task more successfully than an individual effort'. Motivation, creative thinking and brainstorming sessions exist.

2 role clarification
    - Formalization of the network begins with the idea initiator contacting prospective members and arranging a date for the first meeting. 'The idea initiator generally emerges as the group leader and facilitator of group process . . . while members are involved in the group, they do not necessarily believe in the idea of the group' at this stage.

3 negotiation
    - Institutional boundaries are broken and the group works towards common goals and a plan of action is devised. Discussions and relationships continue to develop outside network meetings to form stronger bonds.

4 integration
    - By integrating, Hunt et al. say 'a group personality or code emerges'. The network becomes a cohesive and productive group. Goals are achieved creating the need for a strategic approach for the network. At this stage chairperson, secretary or treasurer may need to be elected. This in turn, demonstrates members believe in the purpose and value of the network.

5 creativity
    - Members of the group feel comfortable and begin to 'display creative talents . . . group members may seek out the unique contribution and expertise of individual people . . . group process and productivity is high'. At this stage the group may finally be called a network.

A similar strategy was adopted by Carr (1982) within four stages. The first stage surrounds initiating a network which may develop following new practices or research. Defining the network's mission which ensures the meetings are positive, focused and goal-orientated encompasses the second stage. A work stage follows whereby 'network members should reach an agreement regarding their purpose and begin to identify action steps to reach their goals'. Furthermore, Carr identifies an active leadership style to steer the group at this level. This will be a positive asset in delegating responsibilities to individual group members. The final stage surrounds 'co-ordination with the professional organization', with both parties gaining benefit. This process allows a professional body to provide financial support and wider access to practitioners. Meanwhile, the network can support an organization's 'efforts in reaching more general goals'.

More recently, Kitson (1993) and Weir and Kendrick (1994) described the process of setting up a network in this country. These works mirror the developing process defined by Carr (1982) and Hunt et al. (1983). These and similar networks have identified a strategic framework from which their groups operate to ensure continued progress.

Recipe for success

The success of any network lies within clearly defined goals and identified ways of achieving them. 'Networking is a give and take process ... successful networkers identify their assets and potentials and recognise their value for others' (O'Connor, 1982). It is a reciprocal process whereby each member contributes unique vital ingredients within a supportive and sharing environment. As Puetz (1983) says, 'in return for information or assistance from others, we help others by serving as a contact for them'. Both Puetz (1983) and Umiker (1989) cite information giving, feedback and developing new contacts or opportunities as the central benefits of networking.

Reaching out and inviting others to become involved is time consuming but essential to the networking process (O'Connor, 1982). The rewards and benefits which result from communicating, sharing and exchanging ideas cannot be over estimated. Within this context Puetz (1983) highlights honesty as being the best policy for prospective networkers. Honesty regarding one's 'skills and abilities' is paramount, as is trust and respect for all members within the group.

Certain rules can be applied when setting up a formal network and Kitson (1993) offers guidelines for this framework:

Do's
- wait for the right time;
- agree on – a philosophy, aims/objectives, organization and finance;
- carefully select steering committee and check their commitment;
- go for the cascade effect, pushing activity and responsibility to others;
- thank people for their help.

Don'ts
- try to speed things up;

- elect all your friends to the steering committee;
- use other network's philosophies or aims;
- tell others what to do;
- expect anything without being prepared to put something into the network.

Pitfalls within networking

Many nurses are reluctant to ask for advice or support within the clinical area. In the past, nurses have been socialized towards an independent task approach to care giving. Nevertheless, the more interdependent style adopted within the present climate represents a competent and holistic approach which encourages a networking philosophy (Umiker, 1989). For many nurses the idea of discussing and debating nursing issues in this way is new and exposure needs encouragement.

Lack of time and both physical and financial resources are challenges for any network. If these can be overcome in the initial stages it offers a foundation on which to plan ahead and seek solutions.

These themes have formed the operational basis of many established networks. In the United Kingdom, the King's Fund Nursing Development Network and the Quality Assurance Network (QUAN) within the Royal College of Nursing are both pertinent examples of how such concepts can be successfully applied to the development of nursing and its practitioners. What can emerge from all this is a climate where practitioners feel supported and able to take the initiative in creating and facilitating change.

All of this was echoed in the underpinning ethos of the Department of Health's *Strategy for Nursing* (1989) and *Vision for the Future* (1993); both of these documents throw down a gauntlet to all of us involved in change and development in nursing. If the challenge is to be met then nurses must cross the traditional boundaries which have hindered the sharing and mutual exchange of ideas and grasp the opportunities which networking can offer.

Networking – the challenge

A central element in the *Vision for the Future* (DOH, 1993) is the notion of dissemination; this intrinsically has a bearing on the nature and direction of sharing the information and knowledge which evolves from clinical practice – this is the pivotal thrust of the networking process. In seeking to maintain this momentum, a conference was arranged under the auspices of the Royal Liverpool University Hospital (NHS) Trust to share knowledge and experience relating to new and expanding roles within the organization. The conference was targeted at practitioners, managers and educators who shared a common vision and commitment to the development of nursing practice within Mersey Region.

The main themes supporting the convergence of these like-minded people focused upon four key elements:

- raising the profile of developing clinical practice within the hospital and Mersey Region;
- creating an environment in which quality nursing is a major goal;
- exploring how practice developments can thrive and remain innovative;
- addressing practice development within a business planning framework.

This ignited a groundswell of enthusiasm which gave substance and energy to the development and establishment of a network for nursing practice within the region.

Towards change – the nurse as a catalyst

Following the conference, nurses at the 'grass-roots' of the profession set about seizing the opportunity to develop a network. Its philosophy would underpin the delivery of high quality care with which to meet client needs.

Within 4 months, an inaugural meeting of the Nursing Practice Development Network was arranged for practitioners from a wide selection of organizational settings. Individuals brought them reflective expertise and representation from the acute sector, community, long-stay/rehabilitation, hospice care, independent areas and higher education.

The initial meeting was successful with an abundance of ideas, suggestions and options for the group to consider. Culmination of the meeting focused upon a brainstorming session to identify key issues regarding the establishment of the network. The key themes to emerge at this stage were:

- SUPPORT
- EDUCATION
- NETWORKING
- SHARING
- DEVELOPMENT

Another predominate theme under the umbrella of the these concepts was the EVOLUTIONARY nature of developing practice and this led to the formation of the acronym SENSED. This can be expanded to express the purpose and activity of the group as Supportive, Educational, Network, Sharing, Evolutionary, Development – and so the term IN-SENSED has meaning, essence and focus (*see* Fig. 5.1).

The 'idea initiation' and 'role clarification' described by Hunt et al. (1983) were displayed, with members forging new links and renewing both formal and informal acquaintances following network meetings. Another stage in the evolvement of the network centred upon 'integration'. This encompassed clarifying and defining the group's remit. The group became known to nurses as the Nursing Practice Development Network and devised five main objectives through which to achieve its purpose and can be referred to by the acronym:

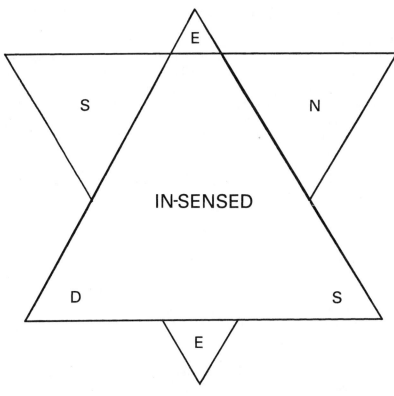

Figure 5.1   IN-SENSED

SUPPORT – supporting and facilitating practitioners in developing research based nursing practice and to assist the evolution of new and expanding roles to meet patient/client needs.

EDUCATION – providing an educational forum for nurses which addresses topical professional issues relating to management, research and practice.

NETWORK – establishing physical links with other practitioners locally, regionally and nationally; and possibly internationally in the future.

SHARING – sharing both knowledge, research and innovations concerning nursing practice development, as a means of promoting access, equality and choice in health care.

EVOLUTIONARY DEVELOPMENT – developing both nurses and nursing practice to create a catalytic process which challenges the boundaries of established practice. This may be achieved in three distinct ways:

- encouraging an ethos of excellence through the practitioner's individual development;
- the continued search for standards of quality in the process of caring;

• facilitating evaluation of care delivery through empowerment and reflection.

By 'integrating', the group was allowed to become 'creative' by seeking ways to operationalize and develop the group within the practice setting. Establishment of a steering group served to facilitate and drive the network creating a foundation upon which to build. The steering group consisted of 12 nurses from practice, education and management backgrounds within the region. A key remit of this group revolved around making the network a proactive resource for all practitioners. As a means of achieving this, an action plan was designed which focused upon the key themes of the network: support, education, sharing and development with specific targets, dates and outcomes. This detailed action plan served to create a framework through which the network could be evaluated after 12 months.

Model for operationalization

The next stage was to address how the network would operate and identify how nurses could benefit from such a local, tangible and challenging resource. A model is intended to give an abstract representation of the framework in which the network operates. This gives a clear indication about the dynamic process of networking.

Structurally, patients/clients, learners and practitioners provide the vital impetus to start the process of networking. The ultimate goals for these people are as follows:

• continuing to develop and deliver research based practice;
• promoting the potential skills of leadership;
• disseminating and sharing clinical expertise to empower both users and providers of nursing (*see* Fig. 5.2).

A scene is set through which a philosophy of networking is exercised. Patients/clients, learners and practitioners bring with them ideas which can lead to the dissemination of information. The identification of needs, problems or challenges can also be highlighted. Once these areas have been identified a rich sense of empowerment and reflection is created through the motivational insights of other individuals. Ultimately, this creates an environment for change (*see* Fig. 5.3).

The process of networking is cyclical in nature as change leads to further reflection and empowerment. Furthermore, developments and innovations challenge the boundaries of nursing practice which may in turn identify new needs and problems.

This is an integral part of the networking process and enables leaders to take an dynamic role as change agents in health care practice. Thus, the dissemination of information and the sharing of ideas is continuous (*see* Fig. 5.4).

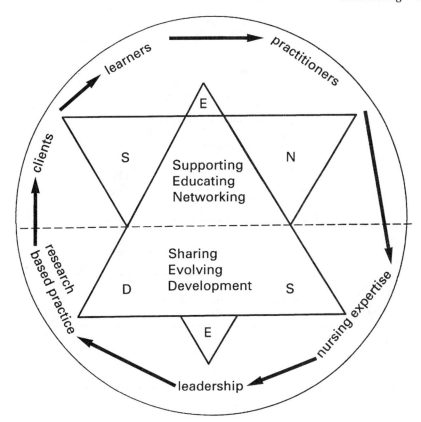

Figure 5.2 Structure of the network

Measuring success

An essential prerequisite for validating the existence of a network lies within the setting of realistic and achievable targets with measurable outcomes. During the early stages of the network's development, a steering group was formed to create an action plan and direct the network to work towards achievable outcomes. Individuals targets were contained in the action plan with reference to the acronym SENSED.

Support

One of the main objectives of any network is to support others. This was true of the Nursing Practice Development Network whose key remit has dealt with supporting and facilitating the development of nursing practice and with it new and

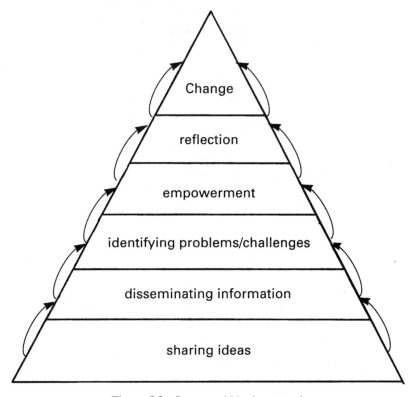

Figure 5.3   Process within the network

expanding roles. The network creates a forum in which to offer direct support to practitioners through link representatives within each trust or unit in the region. This matrix of communication builds in solid foundation for future growth.

Frequent network meetings provide a reciprocal relationship between members of the network and their colleagues in the work place. This channel of communication and feedback enables the network to satisfy ongoing service needs in the clinical area and beyond.

Once individual link people were identified throughout the region, a workshop was arranged whereby these people would meet each other and clarify the role with a view to meeting specific objectives for themselves. The role of link representative within the network has been formalized to incorporate the following remit:

- Present post involves networking within and outside the organization.
- Being an active member of the Nursing Practice Development Network (IN-SENSED).
- Liasing between their unit/organization and the network.
- Providing mutual support and guidance to individual members either by telephone, written correspondence, personal visits and through network meetings.
- Network specific individual area of expertise through acting as a resource.

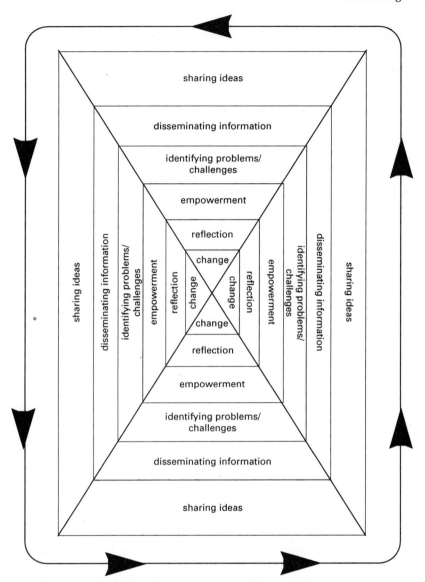

Figure 5.4 Cyclical process

Following the role specification, key objectives essential to this post have been addressed:

- to improve patient care through the discussion and dissemination of nursing practice;
- to update the network with information regarding practice development and ongoing health care research within the unit (yearly);
- to share innovations and developments throughout the Mersey Region via network meetings;

- to provide current information for inclusion in the quarterly newsletter;
- to network throughout organizations and different levels of care delivery (primary, secondary and tertiary) and arrange possible exchange visits, role shadowing and a wide range of other activities;
- to demonstrate, by use of evaluation tools, the benefit to patients of nursing practice developments.

Link representatives are instrumental in promoting and delivering the supportive aspects of the network. This leads us to the second theme within the group's philosophy, that of education and its scope.

Education

The educational aspect inherent within any network can be both vast and widespread. From an early stage, the group identified that an educational remit would be of paramount importance and aimed to provide an educational forum which would address the following issues:

- developing nursing practice;
- recognizing the potential of clinical leadership within the care giving environment;
- promoting and encouraging practice which has been researched and identifies positive, effective outcomes for patient care.

To achieve this end, the educational forum meets quarterly with a varied and structured agenda. The venue for these forums alternates throughout the region and is organized by the link representative who both hosts and chairs the meeting. To date, the educational agendas have discussed and debated current and innovative issues which have direct links with promoting excellence in practice. These have included topics as widespread as the named nurse initiative, risk management, the ethics of networking, research and its application in practice, and patient focused approaches to care delivery within the concepts of both managed care and case management.

The success of the forums is attributed to the link representatives who play a major role at the 'grassroots' in operationalizing the network. Some 30 or 40 practitioners attend these meetings with gusto, eager to share their expertise. The educational forums address both theoretical and practical applications of developments in nursing from a practitioners, managers and academics perspective. This in turn, provides an opportunity for individual and group reflection resulting in much discussion with 'like-minded' health carers.

Networking

At the heart of any network is the networking process. It provides a valuable framework to develop and disseminate new ways in which to practice. With reference to Weir and Kendrick (1994) 'Many practitioners have a reluctance to share their ideas due to the ownership aspect of these innovations. Practitioners are afraid of people "pinching" their ideas and gaining the recognition first. To some, the opportunity to share and support each other is a low priority'. This latter point is particularly relevant in the present internal market of the NHS.

The reluctance to network has hindered many innovators and is something which the Nursing Practice Development Network seeks to remedy. Through networking, links can be made with academic centres enabling bridges to be crossed. The so-called 'theory–practice' gap can be closed as educators and practitioners combine their talents and expertise towards a common goal, that of improving patient care. Through this dual partnership, new opportunities can be exposed to practising nurses. These opportunities centre around being empowered to 'write' for publication in the widest sense. Skills within the higher echelons of academia can facilitate and nurture many budding writers in the clinical area. This reciprocal channel of communication allows nurses to gain credibility and ownership of their innovations and developments through the previously ignored world of writing and publication. Meanwhile, educationalists can update their clinical expertise through the network by reflecting upon patient/client care.

The value of networking cannot be underestimated. With practitioners and educators, educators and managers, managers and practitioners combining forces a truly collaborative, high quality service will ultimately ensue.

Sharing

The sharing aspect of networking is a more tangible and accessible tool for would-be networkers. Sharing ideas and innovations is crucial to the networking process and can be achieved through many avenues.

A quarterly newsletter is freely available to all link representatives which they, in turn, photocopy and distribute throughout their organization, thus incurring minimal costs. Financing any network is a major hurdle and one which we seek to 'share' throughout the region.

Members receive network information concerning recent and forthcoming events via the newsletter which is produced following each educational forum. The theme for each bulletin draws upon the topics which have been the focus of educational seminars.

A written directory of good practice is another example through which sharing excellence in nursing care can be achieved. The network's directory consists of an index of 'good' practice with identified key people who are responsible for the development within their unit; telephone numbers; contact addresses and levels of available support to network members. It is relevant at this point to highlight whether we call these items of good practice either developments, innovations or research and because of this quandary no distinction has been made within the index.

At present, the directory is freely available to all link representatives due to the 'shared' nature of its printing. Individual practitioners submit entries on standardized directory forms which can be easily photocopied and circulated. Not only has this method of distribution been economical, but it has generated a feeling of ownership and partnership within members of the network.

Evolutionary development

Owing to the evolutionary nature of developing practice, the path towards change is continuous and often cyclic. With this, the development of networking nurtures and enables practitioners to become innovative in both their role and in their clinical skills.

The Nursing Practice Development Network continues to grow and develop in both its structure and remit, with the local Mersey Regional Nursing Research Group working closely together with the network. Merging these two groups of practitioners facilitates the change of nursing practice which has been both 'tried and tested'. The incorporation of both research and practice in the same arena will result in positive outcomes for patient care and assist the identification and acceptance of good practice.

The network has been self financing and has survived due to the motivation and enthusiasm of a group of practitioners within a major teaching hospital. They took it upon themselves to create a localized network as a means of fulfilling their roles and promoting nursing practice development within a climate of change. Networking appeared to be integral to their functioning and the freedom to explore such a venture is attributed to the organization in which they work. As developing the network continues to grow from strength to strength, the committed steering group and dedicated link representatives are rewarded with the results.

Striving for excellence

The networking voyage has been one of discovery to say the least. Reflecting on the tidal wave of success seeks to empower the group and motivate others to fulfil a similar need.

At an early stage, the action plan identified targets to attain by an agreed time scale (*see* Tables 5.1–5.5). Achieving these was not without hardship and considerable input by all involved. Surpassing the embryonic stages of its development, the network remains a viable tool through which nurses are enabled to enhance their practice and strive for excellence.

A visionary picture was painted by Weir and Kendrick (1994), who see networking as having 'the potential to encompass interdisciplinary links to promote collaborative working within the primary, secondary and tertiary levels of care delivery'. These views support the new interdependent ethos in care giving which they say 'is the delivery of a co-ordinated and cost effective service which gives informed choice to patient/client, purchaser and provider within the NHS'.

Table 5.1   1994 Target for Action – Support

Objective	Action	Outcomes	Timescale	Responsibility
To support and facilitate the development of nursing practice and the creation of new roles	Direct support will be given through links via representatives within each trust/hospital/unit in the Region	Regular meetings will create a reciprocal relationship between members of the network and their colleagues at their workplace	ONGOING	Link/representatives within each trust/hospital/unit
	Practitioner and patient/client needs can be identified	Ongoing service needs will be met		
	Link representative role clarified and agreed (see Appendix 1)	Role has specific aims and objectives set	Review December 1994	Core group
	Promote co-ordinated seamless care	Link representatives exist within provider and purchasing units	January 1994	
				© IN-SENSED*

* IN-SENSED is the Supportive Educational Network Sharing Evolutionary Development.

Table 5.2 1994 Target for Action – Education

Objective	Action	Outcomes	Timescale	Responsibility
To provide an educational forum which addresses developing nursing expertise; clinical leadership and research based practice	Network members to meet quarterly with structured programme and pro forma guidelines (see Appendix 2)	The educational application of developments in nursing will provide an opportunity for reflection and discussion	FEBRUARY, MAY, AUGUST AND NOVEMBER (Ongoing)	Link representatives to structure meetings, agendas and programmes
	Forum will discuss and debate current and innovate issues which have direct links with promoting excellence in practice (last ½ h of forum)			
	Evaluation forms will be utilized (see Appendix 3)	To steer network	ONGOING	
	Annual conferences organized	Conference takes place within the region	November/December 1994	

© IN-SENSED

Table 5.3   1994 Target for Action – Networking

Objective	Action	Outcomes	Timescale	Responsibility
To establish links with other practitioners locally, regionally and nationally	Networking exists via representatives throughout the region	Official launch of the network via press, radio etc.	Re-publicize November/ December 1994	Core group
	Encourage members to write for publication	Members write articles for professional journals	ONGOING	All members
	Establish links with academic centres	Reduction in theory/ practice gap	ONGOING	All members
	Establish links with publishers	Publication of book entitled *Innovations in Practice*	1994	Editoral panel and contributors
				© IN-SENSED

Table 5.4   1994 Target for Action – Sharing

Objective	Action	Outcomes	Timescale	Responsibility
To share both the knowledge and innovations concerning nursing practice development	Produce a quarterly newsletter following educational forum	Newsletter informs members about recent and forthcoming events; and the progress of the network to date. Contains a list of link/representatives and contact area; and a letter/information column/page	MARCH, JUNE, SEPTEMBER AND DECEMBER, respectively	Member of core group
	A written directory is produced	Directory identifies good practice. A list of telephone numbers, addresses, areas of interest and level of support is available	Revised April 1994	Member of core group
	Newsletter contributions by last day of the month	Newsletter printed	FEBRUARY, MAY, AUGUST AND NOVEMBER respectively	All members
	Database	Database exists and acts as a resource for disseminating and evaluating good practice	To be reviewed	Under discussion

© IN-SENSED

Table 5.5   1994 Target for Action – Evolutionary Development

Objective	Action	Outcomes	Timescale	Responsibility
To develop both nurses and nursing to challenge the boundaries of nursing practice	The growth and remit of the network is formalized	Continued development of the network will assist individual practitioners to be innovative in their role and practice	ONGOING	Core group and representatives
	The network has the potential to undertake research to evaluate nursing practice throughout Region	'Good practice' is identified and accepted	ONGOING	All members
	The network and the Mersey Region Nursing Research Group work closely together	Practice development underpins research findings	ONGOING	Core group and link representatives
				© IN-SENSED

Art of networking

Within the literature, numerous articles have discussed and debated the beneficial aspects of networking. The concept is not new, exclusive or out of reach for any-one who wants to utilize the process. However, Christy (1987), in referring to the work of Puetz (1983), identifies several 'rules of thumb':

* keeping in touch with contacts;
* sharing information which is useful for others;
* being honest;
* do not ask people or yourself to do things you know you or they are not capable of doing;
* do not burn your 'bridges'.

However, Hurff et al. (1990) continue this theme with the following:

* keep the network focused;
* communicate frequently;
* keep it small;
* keep it simple and cheap;
* remember the reciprocal relationship.

A network offers opportunities to share. Sharing offers opportunities for education. Education offers opportunities for networking. Networking offers opportunities to give support. Supporting one another enables practitioners to develop and evolve new ways to deliver nursing practice. This is explicit within the Nursing Practice Development Network as it uses the acronym IN-SENSED to steer and drive the group.

Finally, in the words of McCray (1986): 'Through the formation of networks and coalitions we gain the necessary strength and momentum to positively influence health care policy. Although the goal seems large, when each of us is willing to assume responsibility in our own personal sphere of influence, collectively our strength and influence cannot be ignored'.

References

Anderson R, Pierce I, Ringl K (1983) Networking: a method of retaining nursing staff. *Journal of Nursing Administration*; **12** [9(2)]: 26–28.

Carr EM (1982) Networking: a resource for change. *Nurse Practitioner*; **7**: 32–34.

Christy KA (1987) Networks: forming 'old-girls' connections among nurses. *Nursing Management*; **18** [4]: 73–75.

Concise Oxford English Dictionary (1990) *Concise Oxford English Dictionary*, 8th Edition. Oxford: Oxford University Press.

DOH (1989) *Strategy For Nursing*. A Report of the Steering Committee. London: HMSO.

DOH (1993) *Vision for the Future*. The Nursing, Midwifery and Health Visiting Contribution to Health and Health Care NHS Management Executive. London: HMSO.

Fain J, Viau P (1989) Networking: A strategy for strengthing the role of the clinical nurse specialist. *Clinical Nurse Specialist*; **3** [1]: 29–31.

Ferguson M (1980) *The Aquarian Conspiracy.* Los Angeles: JP Tarcher.

Harter C, Grossman LK, Swank E, Spring B (1989) Networking to implement effective health care. *American Journal of Maternal Child Nursing*; **14** [6]: 387–392.

Hockenbery-Eaton M (1992) Nursing research – moving forward through networking. Collaboration and mentorship. *Journal Of Paediatric Oncology*; **9** [3]: 132–135.

Hunt V, Stark JL, Fisher F, Hegedus K, Joy L, Woldum K (1983) Networking: A managerial strategy for research revelopment in a service setting. *Journal of Nursing Administration.* July/August; **13**: 31–32.

Hurff JM, Lowe HE, Ho BJ, Hoffman NM (1990) Networking: a successful linkage for community occupational therapists. *American Journal Of Occupational Therapy.* May; **14** [5]: 424–430.

Kitson A (1993) Setting up a network. *Nursing Standard*; **7** [27]: 7–8.

Lynch E (1993) Organisational networking empowerment through politics. In: Marriner-Tomey A, (ed.), *Transformational Leadership In Nursing.* Chapter 12. Chicago: Mosby-Year Book.

Mackereth PA, Sheenan A, Wright SG (1994) A vision for the future. Part 2: Targets 5–9. *Nursing Standard*; **8** [50]: 29–32.

McCray N (1986) Networks and coalitions: tools for strength. *Oncology Nursing Forum*; **13** [4]: July/August 103–104.

McKendrick J (1982) The role of networking. *Management World*; **11** [2]: 21.

Meisenhelder JB (1982) Networking and nursing. *Image*; **14** [3] October: 77–80.

Murphy JK (1988) Networking across professional lines. *Paediatric Nursing* March/April 1988; **14** [2]: 133–134.

O'Connor AB (1982) Ingredients for successful networking. *Nurse Educator* Winter 1982; **14** [6]: 40–43.

Puetz BE (1983) Is networking for you? *Occupational Health Nursing*; **31** June: 34–37.

Smith, MJ (1987/8) Valuing – A key to networking quality nursing. *Nursing Forum*; **23** [2]: 56–59.

Umiker W (1989) Networking: A vital activity for health care professionals. *Health Care Supervisor*; **7** [3]: 65–69.

Wake M, Vogel G (1985) Networking: reducing competition while increasing collegiality. *Dimensions of Critical Care Nursing*; **4** [3]: 132–134.

Weir P, Kendrick K (1994) Setting up networks to improve practice. *Nursing Standard*; **8** [41]: 29–33.

Wright S (1990) *Changing Nursing Practice.* London: Edward Arnold.

6 Facilitating action learning in nursing: does the hand fit the glove?

Elaine Rosser

> We do not learn by doing . . . we learn by doing and realizing what came of what we did.
>
> (Dewey, 1929)

Rote learning, or rather learning in sequence with little or no relevance to the practical application of what was learned, was viewed as the most successful method of acquiring knowledge up until the 1930s. In 1938 Revans both challenged and questioned such an approach, (Lessem, 1991). He presented the view that, for people to learn productively and effectively, they need to learn by doing and then reflecting on their actions. He called this process Action Learning. On further consideration, it can be seen also as an empowering tool for individuals, giving them a choice of how they meet the demands and stresses of the world, whether actively or passively (Morgan and Ramirez, 1984). It enables people to see how learning occurs through past and current experiences. An interesting perception of it is explored by Ali Khan (1991). She relates it to a 'green' form of learning, one that can even influence social systems. Action learning involves the challenging of hidden assumptions, and the changing of methods of work, social patterns, and management styles.

Action learning is not an easy option or a quick fix development. The question is: will the nursing development hand fit the action learning glove? The flexibility of action learning could work in tandem with the 'roaring current' of change within the National Health Service (NHS), particularly within nursing, (Toffler, 1973). It could be a powerful instrument to help nursing meet the challenges of the twentieth century and beyond (DOH, 1993). It is certain that nowadays nurses, educationalists, and organizations (particularly the NHS) need to develop the skill of lateral thinking (De Bono, 1967). We live in an 'upside-down world' (Handy, 1991), and need theory linked to practice and practice linked to theory in order to survive. It is important to see action learning as a whole, not with its various aspects in separate compartments. Each part is linked to every other, in a cyclical process, because of the doing, reflecting, facilitating, and questioning elements of the method.

This chapter is an exploration – through a review of current literature and the use of case studies – of the efficiency, effectiveness, and relevance of action learning to nursing. This has to be seen as not only a tool to develop nurses and nursing professionally, but also as something vital to an organization's growth.

People do have their own preferred learning styles. They know, or think they know, how they learn best and where their strengths and development needs lie. However, in order to move forward, it is sometimes necessary to challenge our most comfortable assumptions, to develop something that at first glance appears risky. Action learning offers the chance to do this, and it offers it in a supportive and constructive environment. Having said that, it is important to stress that it is not for everyone: individual learning needs are always to be respected and even anticipated.

The doing part (having an experience)

The doing part of the cyclical process of action learning can also be called having an experience. The participants work on real cases, and they learn from each other through questioning, challenging, and mutual support. They are committed to the completion of their task, wherever possible. Peters and Waterman (1982) describe someone who works on a task and learns from it as a 'project champion'. It is, of course, necessary to have had an experience to be able to reflect, plan, and act on it. Perhaps the hardest part of this is being able to recognize the experience and be comfortable with the self-awareness it evokes. According to Boyd and Fales (1983),'the outcome of the process is a changed conceptual perspective'.

The following case study describes how an action learning set can evolve.

Case study 1

Mary worked within the Development and Training Department of a large teaching hospital. She had recently read an article about the benefits to an organization of action learning, and she was interested in using this method of learning with ward managers. Mary was a pragmatist and she could see its application to practice. However, she was unsure of how to make the idea a successful reality. She recognized that she had an inadequate understanding of the process. She therefore decided to review the current literature and establish in her own mind precisely how action learning would benefit her organization and the ward managers. She identified her need to seek out someone with the relevant experience to help her, and she decided to approach her manager who, she knew, had facilitated an action learning set. Mary drew up a list of questions to ask her.

Key questions Mary asked

1 What is the definition of action learning?
2 What is an action learning set?
3 How large is a set?
4 Who nominates the set members?
5 What is a set adviser?

6   How should she evaluate action learning's efficiency, effectiveness, and relevance in relation to her organization?

Practical application

Mary's manager explained to her that action learning was the name given to learning through action. It was a continuous process that helped people to deal with life's problems. She said: 'Action learning builds on this normal process of learning, making the links more clear in order to make them effective' (McGill and Beaty, 1993).

She said that a set consists simply of people who want to be involved in action learning. There is no hierarchical structure within a set, unless its members establish one themselves. The set is encouraged to work in partnership, sharing with each other and supporting and encouraging each other.

The size of a set is usually six to eight people. If it were bigger it would be unable to have the time to meet the individual needs of each set member. The length of a set's life is normally 9 months, but this can vary from set to set. The closing of a set is based on a decision made by the set members, not the set adviser.

Mary's manager emphasized that people must nominate themselves if they wish to be set members. This is because not everyone likes or feels comfortable with this form of learning. Nevertheless, it is surprising how often people are willing to break away from their established way of doing things, when they need help to approach and deal with an issue that has proved hard to resolve.

Mary's manager defined the set adviser as the group's facilitator. This person plays a key role in observing the group process and channelling the group in the right direction. Handy (1991) describes some jobs as like doughnuts! The jam in the middle represents the part of the job that is clearly defined, and the other part of the 'doughnut' is the unclear and fuzzy area of the role that requires developing. In some ways this is not a bad definition.

In these days of cost effectiveness, the appropriate use of resources, and value for money, it is worth highlighting that people are a valued yet frequently underused asset to an organization. If a new method of learning is to be used, it must be clearly defined and the benefits to the individual and the workplace must be linked to the satisfaction of corporate needs.

The evaluation of the effectiveness, efficiency, and relevance of action learning can best be understood in its processes. Mary's manager explained that it offers the individual a rate of learning that tends to be greater than the rate of change in the environment (Garrett, 1987). This is the reason why it has proved successful and been well used in the NHS (Morse, 1991). It offers the scope to blend personal, organizational, and group needs into a cohesive structured system that benefits all. In the past, courses have given participants the knowledge they needed, but not the framework to help them to develop the knowledge acquired into a competency. According to Swieringa and Wierdsma (1992), action learning offers such a framework.

In 1986, Morris stated that 'the acid test of effective investment in learning is whether the learning can be applied'. Historically, training has been evaluated only on the trainer's reputation. Today's climate places an emphasis on evaluating training in the light of a participant's behaviour changes and increased effectiveness within the workplace. This usually leads to effective resource management.

In 1986, Bramley cited five purposes of training evaluation: feedback, control, research intervention, and power games. Feedback evaluation takes account of the changes in the behaviour of the participant. Control evaluation is concerned with the linking of training and development to the policy and practice of the emphasis on value for money in an organization. Research evaluation brings the training knowledge into the practice. Intervention evaluation is about the analysis of the training needs of an organization. Power games evaluation focuses on the misuse of power games.

From all this, we can see that there is no single right or set way to evaluate action learning. Its success lies in the understanding and commitment of the participants and the relevance of the process to the real life issues which they face.

At the end of their interview, Mary's manager gave her a word of warning about being a set adviser. The set adviser must enable action learning to occur and must possess specific attributes: patience, courage, self-awareness, the ability to observe the set process, tolerance, and a willingness to challenge and support the group. These attributes will be explored in detail in the next case study.

The reflecting (reviewing the experience)

Learning from an experience requires a review of what went well and what could have been done better. This reviewing stage is an on-going part of action learning and integral to its success.

The participants learn from each other and question and challenge each other's problems, results, and ideas. It is not an exaggeration to say that the result of this process can sometimes be likened to being born again, so great is the power of its questioning approach to overturn views and perceptions once thought to be unshakable.

Reflection, evaluation, and feedback can occur at different stages in the life of the set. They can occur at the beginning of a group's meeting, during it, and at the end. Sometimes matters are left for several weeks and then reviewed, depending on the specific needs of each individual set.

McGill and Beaty (1993) give a list of headings to show ways in which reviewing and reflection are likely to occur:

- One thing that I have gained from being in the set today.
- One thing I have gained/learned about the way the set works.
- Something I would like the set to consider that I am not yet sure about.
- Something I want to share that I have difficulty with when I am presenting and/or when I am a set member giving support to another.

- Something I want to say about the set, myself, the set adviser, another set member.

Case study 2

Henry was a set adviser for an action learning set of newly qualified staff nurses. The set had been established for 6 months, and in that time the group had become supportive and productive, and the individual needs of each member were valued.

At the last couple of meetings Henry had sensed a dramatic change in the group dynamics. Two members of the set, Janet and Frank, were openly critical of each other and appeared to be working in fierce competition with each other. The other set members found this situation uncomfortable and harmful to the life of the set.

Initially, Henry had decided not to interfere with Janet's and Frank's behaviour, but to observe the processes of group reaction. He hoped the set members would regulate the situation themselves.

Matters came to a head at a meeting where Helen, another set member, was presenting an unusual and challenging issue. It was her specific 'time' with the set. Janet and Frank openly ignored Helen's issue and took over her 'speak' time to compete against each other. Henry sensed the group's despondency, frustration, and anger at this treatment of Helen by Frank and Janet.

Henry stopped the group and asked them to feedback on how they were feeling within the group now. The feedback was as Henry had suspected: they felt angry and aggressive towards Janet and Frank for their treatment of Helen. The group felt that Janet and Frank had broken two of the initial ground rules of the group, by not valuing each other's opinions and not respecting someone else's time to speak without interruption.

Janet and Frank were surprised at the group's feelings. The group decided to review their ground rules and find out what had gone wrong.

Key questions Henry needed to address in this situation

1 What was the reason for Janet and Frank's behaviour?
2 How was the situation affecting the group process, and is this situation normal in group life?
3 What role should Henry play as set adviser in acknowledging and resolving the situation?

Practical application

Henry needed to explore, either inside or outside the group, why Janet and Frank were in opposition to each other. They needed to be made aware of their actions and of their lack of productivity. A solution or compromise needed to be found. The members of the action learning group are the prime sources of help more often than the set adviser.

Such a stormy period is normal in group life and is healthy. However, the problem has to be challenged. Unchallenged, it can destroy group productivity and support. The problem keeps the group alive and developing, and enables it to be alert to situations that must be addressed. The despondency and anger of the group at the situation, which Henry sensed so strongly, needed challenging and channelling into positive outcomes.

Henry, as set adviser, made the group aware of the issue in a safe environment. He gave them the opportunity to explore and find solutions to what was happening. The use of the established group rules aided this process. This is all part of the group's learning and enhances their development.

The role of the set adviser

A set adviser must be clear about a role before facilitating a set, as understanding of the role is crucial to the success of the set.

The quality of genuineness in the set adviser, as identified by Rogers (1979), is so important that it must be mentioned first. It must not be forgotten that the uniqueness of a set is achieved through the personality of the set adviser as much as through the set members.

The set adviser needs to move from the traditional teacher's role and reskill himself/herself. As happens with the participants, old skills are lost and new skills are learned. The process can be compared to a birth and the pain and joy that are associated with birth.

The adviser has five important functions within the set. They are: facilitating, giving, receiving, clarifying group processes, and enabling the group to be self-functioning (Casey, 1991). Each function appears at a different time in the life of the set. The set adviser needs enough maturity and self-awareness to feel comfortable with letting the group self-function. To give away for a time what has become part of you is hard, but the success of the adviser and the set often depends upon this giving.

In the previous case study, Henry needed to be skilful in the timing of his intervention relating to Janet's and Frank's behaviour. He asked painful, challenging, and open, but supportive questions. The adviser forces people to face the toughness of reality 'by doing U-turns, reversals and full stops' (Lawlor, 1991).

A set has been described as a real life laboratory where feedback comes from four main sources and is immediate (Lawlor, 1991). These four sources are: the set, set advisers, clients, and review points. The set members are well placed to give open constructive feedback. The set advisers provide the enabling part of the feedback, achieving this through encouragement, the taking of personal risks, and intuitiveness. The clients are the people – that is peers, subordinates, or supervisors – who play a key role in the reflections of each set member; they may be a part of the task that needs addressing. The review points are the structures that allow feedback to occur: without the acknowledgement of feedback times it cannot happen.

Henry needed to use his skill to say nothing and appear invisible as appropriate. He had to take a personal risk when the group did not handle the situation and address it openly. This is part of the courage of the set adviser, which enables him to tread on territory not yet conquered. The set adviser is not in a traditional teacher role whereby the pupil listens and learns from the teacher. Here the teacher is a learner too. Skills and knowledge are used to help the learner to understand better, and this is achieved by group support.

The most exciting and rewarding part of the set adviser's role is when the group begins to move together, support each other, and solve real cases. In the author's own experience it is like a journey and the feeling of elation you have when eventually you arrive at your destination after several delays and detours.

Theories of change relating to action learning

Theories of change settle well into the description of a group's life. There are, according to Lewin (1958), three stages: unfreezing, moving, and refreezing. Unfreezing is where the need for change occurs and established norms are reviewed. Moving is sought from participants to help with the change. Refreezing is when the change becomes firmly established and integrated. For change to be effective, this last stage has to occur. Lewin also looked at the forces that aid and prevent change occurring. To initiate a change all the stages must be planned and a change agent identified.

There are many strategies to effect a change, and three major ones were identified by Bennis et al. (1976): rational empirical, power coercive, and normative re-educative. The rational empirical strategy is based on the belief that if someone is given the facts, sound reason will prevail. The power coercive strategy stresses force as a method of change. Meanwhile, the normative re-educative strategy stresses the need for knowledge, education, and support in change. Each change agent should adopt the method appropriate to the change required (Wright, 1989).

Group processes

This area of development is fascinating and stimulating. It is interesting to see how the account above of case study 2 shows a group proceeding through the four stages in a group's life as defined by Tuckman (1965): forming, storming, norming, and performing. Of course, a group can move backwards as well as forwards in these stages of its life, and sometimes (as the above case study shows) it can move backwards in order to take a greater leap forwards.

Hunt (1979) has described five phases in the influence of individual behaviour on a group as a whole.

Phase one

This is the initial period of tolerance. Deviation by members of the group is noted, and the group members seek an explanation and make excuses for the situation.

Phase two

The members of the group make an open attempt to resolve the deviation and correct the behaviour they dislike. At this stage the members are not tolerating the situation, and they signal verbally and non-verbally that it must stop.

Phase three

The members of the group become angry. They may even become verbally aggressive.

Phase four

At this stage physical aggression can occur.

Phase five

The individual deviant within the group is asked to leave. Once this occurs, the group balances its roles again and the life of the group recommences. Silence is often used as a means of rejection. However, silence can also be welcomed as giving a period of peace and reflection.

It needs to be highlighted here that not all of these five phases occur in sequence, if they occur at all.

Conflict has more than one side to it. If constructive, it can energize group relationships (Hunt, 1979). On the other hand, destructive conflict is injurious to the social system.

Styles of learning

According to Kolb (1984), the experiential model of learning is closely related to the cycle of action learning: it mirrors it. Meanwhile, Honey (1986) identifies through an 80-item questionnaire learning styles linked to attributes of individual people. These may be expressed as follows:

- The activist is game for anything new (case studies 1 and 4).
- The reflector likes to take time to ponder an issue or situation (case studies 2 and 3).
- The theorist relates issues to theories and how they work (case studies 2 and 4).
- The pragmatist is always asking the question: how can I apply this in practice? (case study 1).

When a teacher is identifying learning for an individual, it is necessary to link it wherever possible to the individual's preferred learning style.

The facilitating

Proficiency in this skill requires experience and natural talent. Involved in a major Canadian scheme, Morgan (1988) identified the competences that managers and senior executives need in order to work in our 'upside down' world. These are: viewing people as your main asset and resource, flattering hierarchical structures, allowing facilitation and networking to occur, and developing and sharing real cases while providing the support and advice to resolve them. In summary, he sees the skills of active facilitation as managing the group process by adopting 'a reflective synthesizing approach to group discussion . . . interventions that frame and reframe the issues . . . making an unobtrusive record of the group discussion'.

The framing and reframing of issues requires clarity to emphasize the necessity and value of it. This is when the set adviser or a set member places a case in its current context, thus clarifying hidden issues or misunderstandings by the group. Sometimes it is a case of saying, openly, what the group wanted to say.

Facilitation allows empowerment, energizing, and openness to occur (case studies 2, 3 and 4).

Case study 3

Ann had been a member of her action learning set for 9 months. The set was in the process of ending. Ann had found her fellow set members invaluable in their support and knowledge. She had been able to resolve many key issues, and her development needs were consistently addressed and met.

Reflecting on where she had been and where she now was gave Ann much pleasure. To be able to reflect positively on a learning experience was new to Ann. Initially, self and group feedback had been hard. Now it had become a way of life to her, and she valued it.

One of her colleagues, Jack, approached her with an interest in reflection. He was unsure how it worked, but he wanted to understand it. Ann considered how she should begin to help him.

Key questions Ann needs to address

1   How would she define reflection for Jack?
2   What role does reflection play in an individual's learning experience?
3   How can one analyse and place reflection in a developmental programme?
4   Who supports the results of one's reflection?

Practical application

Ann used the definition of Boyd and Fales (1983) to define the meaning of reflection to Jack. They view reflection as 'the process of creating and clarifying the means of experience (present or past) in terms of self (self in relation to self and self in relation to the world).' They state that it is not a new concept, but rather a natural process.

People's self-confidence increases when they are exposed to talking and reflecting on the uncertainties of situations (Garrett, 1991). Identifying the need to reflect by doing, rather than simply by thinking retrospectively, can make experiences alive and relatable (Schon, 1983).

Ann explored with Jack the self-awareness that reflection involves. This raised self-awareness fulfils some development needs and prevents the stagnation of ideas. There are a 'true' and a 'false' self, according to Laing (1959). The 'true' self is one's inner private self, while the 'false' self is one's pretending, outer self. There is also a simpler model of the self in which it consists of three domains – thoughts, feelings, and behaviour – with all of them interlinked (Burnard, 1990).

Ann talked to Jack also about the need for appropriate support in order to understand what is being reflected upon, how to learn from it, and what to do to move forward. Unsupported reflection can be a lonely, disturbing, and painful process. Supported, it can still at times be disturbing and painful, but strategies can be suggested to deal with these feelings. Properly supported reflection can open windows, show new opportunities, and provide a catalyst for personal change and development. It allows the therapeutic use of oneself.

The questioning

Questions are simple, easy to ask, and easy to answer? That is very far from the truth! If people never asked questions the world would be a boring and predictable place to live in. The vitality of a set depends on the intensity, relevance, and clarity of the questions that are asked. Questions may be open or probing or closed. An open question gives the person questioned the opportunity to answer fully and explore a variety of ideas and responses. An example would be 'Can you tell me the problem you have brought to this set?' A probing question may be exemplified by 'Can you clarify what you mean by saying you feel uncomfortable in the group?' A closed question allows for no exploration or probing; for example, 'How long have you been a member of this set?'.

It is appropriate at this point to explore leadership and questioning and their relationship to action learning.

Leadership and action learning

Good leadership is crucial to the successful development of any organization (Swieringa and Wierdsma, 1992). Good leaders have the ability to utilize people's expertise for the good of all. The ability to involve, include, and empower people as a leadership strategy is termed 'shared governance' (Neis and Kingdon, 1990). There are four basic leadership styles: directing, coaching, supporting, and delegating. Action learning can be a way of using the supporting style to produce high calibre leaders.

There is a question mark over nursing's ability to promote a leadership culture, according to Rafferty (1993). In an interview study she identifies two key themes: 'leadership as a constellation of attributes and qualities and leadership as a process of managing and influencing change'. These can both be seen in the role of the set adviser.

From another point of view, there are two distinct forms of leadership: visible and charismatic, and less visible. Initially, Henry in case study 2 adopted the latter approach. There is a close link between leadership and change, as Adair (1988) has noticed. Good leaders see the need and implement the change when others ignore or do not even see the need. Henry saw that it was necessary to focus the group on its problems, becoming in the process more visible himself, when invisibility had proved unsuccessful as a method. In being open to the group about the issues that had to be faced, Henry showed his courage. He could have been used as a scapegoat for the group's problems. He took the risk.

Strong leaders show the way and create a vision which shows people how they can deal with change (Kanter, 1990). This strong sense of direction and this vision empower people to make progress. Mary and Diane (case studies 1 and 4) displayed these qualities. They knew where they wanted to go, and sought the appropriate person and information to enable them to plan the journey. Henry (case study 2) realized his set were losing direction, and focused their attention on a way of solving their problems and moving forward. Kanter's definition of leadership fits well within the strategic thinking of an organization, and it allows for 'a change process that is deliberate and conscious articulation of a direction'.

Leadership strategies that deal with change within an organization 'harness the most immediate and accessible source of knowledge and power: the aggregate intellect and expertise of their people' (Neis and Kingdon, 1990). People are a leader's and organization's greatest asset, and action learning is all about valuing people and supporting them to develop personally and professionally.

In case study 4 some of the processes of action learning are used to develop leadership skills.

Case study 4

Diane was asked by her Director of Nursing Services to facilitate a group of clinical leaders within her hospital. Diane saw the doing, reflecting, and reviewing components of action learning as some ways of making the group supportive and challenging to each other and enabling them to address their individual and group needs.

At the first meeting Diane explained to the group how these processes could be used by the clinical leaders. She was aware of some reservations expressed by the group: they were unsure what action learning was and what these processes were. Diane explained to the group that they would not be an action learning set in the true sense; but the process of action learning – doing, reflecting, and reviewing – would provide useful strategies for them as clinical leaders. She suggested they might 'try it and see what happens' for a trial period of 4 months. The group agreed.

Throughout this period, Diane played a strong role in advising the group on how to use these strategies. She used the five headings listed by McGill and Beaty (1993) in connection with reflection and reviewing. This assisted the clinical leaders to centralize their tasks and provide results in their roles, which was fundamental to the value and future of their roles in the organization.

When the 4-month trial period finished, Diane discussed the results with the group.

Key questions Diane addressed

1 How successful did the group and individuals feel the progress had been?
2 Had any achievements been evaluated?
3 Did this method of learning lend itself to their needs and the needs of their organization?

Practical application

Initially, the group members had to think closely about the progress made. They found it easier to analyse their own individual progress than the overall success of the group. Diane explored with them the stages of group forming that they had gone through (Tuckman, 1965), and they were fascinated to see how they had fitted into this group theory. Diane helped them to reflect on the initial issues they had brought to the group and how the group had helped them to move forward.

They had already evaluated their individual achievements by observing the impact they had had on their own areas. They mentioned how their staff had commented on their improved technique in problem solving and their greater regard for the value of team work.

Finally, Diane asked them whether they saw the components of action learning as responsive to the needs of an individual in a changing organization. They replied that the strategies used in action learning were adaptable and useful for deciding on a clear direction in a world of change.

What is a learning organization?

'Essentially, learning organizations are not only capable of learning, but also of learning to learn. In other words, they are not only able to become competent, but also to remain competent' (Swieringa and Wierdsma, 1992).

Action learning fits like a glove on the hand of a learning organization. It is adaptable to the changing needs involved. It also facilitates the organization's movement in the direction it wants to take, through structural questioning and the challenging of motives. Development can be seen as the ability to adapt without losing identity (Swieringa and Wierdsma, 1992).

Development is a key concept in a learning organization, in that the learning process is problem orientated. Problems clarify who needs to be involved and what needs to be learned in order to resolve the problems. Problem orientated learning is cyclical and fits neatly within the framework of action learning, which involves doing, reflecting, facilitating and questioning. In a learning organization, doing and questioning cannot be seen as separate, and they need to be linked to reflection and decision making. All this can be collective and occur in teams. Work in teams can form the basis for the fulfilment of the potential for self-knowledge, especially knowledge of how and why you are learning and what you wish to learn.

Why become a learning organization?

An organization needs to be constantly learning in order to deal with rapid change and so survive. Increased emphasis is now placed on research, development, service, and consultancy.

The Trekker model for a learning organization is interesting (Swieringa and Wierdsma, 1992). In this model changes occur which cause people not to know precisely where they are heading and where they will finish up. We choose the direction and off we go! With this type of approach the process of re-organization and the behavourial changes are integrated. If we knew how to cope with the unknown, we would perform better. According to Lawlor (1991), an advantage of action learning is that it saves cost because the worker is learning on the job. Lawlor describes it in this way:

> Managers are discovering that they can find the time to deal with their real problems and at the same time contend with the alligators that have been diverting their energies away from draining the swamp.

The diversity of organizational styles combines well with the flexibility of action learning. The key to its success is that it does not pretend that there is only one right approach to any problem. Action learning meets the needs of the organization, rather than the organization meeting the needs of action learning!

Evaluating action learning

There is an abundance of definitions of the word evaluation, as Easterby-Smith and Burgoyne (1991) are keen to stress. They discuss two of these definitions: evaluation as judgement, and evaluation as development. The former sees evaluation as a means of assessing the quality and worth of the training offered; the latter sees evaluation as a preliminary to improving a planned programme.

Analysis of the success of action learning can be difficult. This is because of the different contexts in which the set members work, and the different approaches they use. Nevertheless, we may reasonably see it as a useful tool to help an organization survive as it experiences changes. Baker (1980) in McLean and Marshall (1988) sees it as a way of preventing employees and employers getting stuck in 'the social glue that holds the organization together'. This glue can stifle and destroy cultural change and creativity.

In evaluating action learning, it is vital to be aware of why this method was used and what problems were seen as likely to be encountered.

How to plan an action learning set. Key steps to take

1   Plan a literature review of action learning. Focus on examples of action learning occurring in your own area of practice. The reader may well find it of benefit here to refer to the works of Reginald Revans (1983) and Mike Pedlar (1991).
2   Establish a definition of action learning and decide how it will fit into your organizational specifications.
3   Identify the key skills of a set adviser. Seek training in these skills from an experienced set adviser who may act as a mentor and help you to reflect and to self-regulate your behaviour as appropriate. There are, for instance, times when it is necessary to be 'invisible' within a group, and this form of verbal restraint can be demanding. It is worth remembering that the support and challenging which the set adviser needs will be provided by the group.
4   Understand the stages of group formation that will be an integral part of set life.
5   Identify the members of the set through their self-nomination.
6   Decide on the times of meetings, the venues, and the agendas.
7   The group must establish ground rules and agree on the function and role of the set adviser.
8   Observe continually the group as a whole and each member individually. Highlight to the group the process which is occurring as the situation may require.
9   The process, workings, and evaluation of the group are identified and explored at each set meeting.
10 Time must be allocated at different set meetings for a set member to present a particular issue for discussion.
11 How do we end the life of a set? The normal lifespan of a set is 9 months, but it can vary. The decision to end a set is not made by the set adviser, but is part of a natural progression in its usefulness to the members. This can be a sad phase; but it can also be valuable in displaying the learning curves that the group has progressed through. The ending of a set can be viewed as a new beginning. Many members of an action learning set go on to become set

advisers; indeed, such membership is usually a necessary preliminary to becoming an adviser.

Problems to be encountered with action learning

1 Anything at all may be said within the group, and it is obvious how difficult or embarrassing that can be.
2 Group members who dominate the speaking time of the set will have to be challenged.
3 Group members may be manipulated to abuse the safety and confidentiality of the group.
4 This is not an easy method of learning.
5 There may be a lack of organizational commitment to action learning.
6 Some set members may not be fully committed to action learning.
7 The facilitator may be inexperienced.
8 The set adviser may fail to let go and allow the group to self-facilitate.
9 There may be a failure to end the set when the group processes are highlighting the end.
10 There may be no established ground rules agreed by the set.
11 Time may not be given for reflection, review, and evaluation.

Wearing the glove

Many facets of action learning have been explored. Its dynamic cyclical processes lend themselves to the changing needs of the nursing profession and the NHS. It fosters the creativity of an organization through the diverse and flexible approaches which it makes possible (Morgan and Ramirez, 1984; Morgan, 1988).

Reflection, problem solving, and decision making are central to its processes, and they prevent the individual and the organization from falling in with 'the alligators in the swamp' (Lawlor, 1991), and being 'stuck in the social glue', (Baker, 1980; McLean and Marshall, 1988).

Action learning generates the belief within individuals and organizations that learning can help you change your behaviour and fulfil your identified goals. There are many studies which stress that those organizations where staff are valued, supported, and allowed to grow and innovate are the most successful (Orton, 1981; McClure et al., 1983).

However, a word of caution! Action learning is not a cure for all ills. It has to be carefully analysed before being used, since we must be clear on why we want to use it. The glove of action learning can fit the hand of nursing just so long as we ensure we have the right glove size.

We do control the future . . . We can wait, react . . . and reel from the changes around us, or we can seize the opportunity and ride the surf!

IT'S YOUR ROAD, YOUR FUTURE!
(Neis and Kingdon, 1990)

References

Adair J (1988) *The Action-Centred Leader.* Guildford and King's Lynn: Biddles.

Ali Khan S (1991) Action learning is 'green'. In: McGill I, Beaty L (eds), *Action Learning. A Practitioner's Guide.* London: Kogan Page, pp 224–225.

Baker E (1980) Managing organisational culture. In: McLean A, Marshall J (eds) (1988), *Cultures at Work. How to Identify and Understand Them.* Luton: Local Government Training Board, 2.

Bennis WG, Benne KD, Chin R, Corey KE (1976) *The Planning of Change.* London: Holt Rinehart and Winston.

Boyd EM, Fales AW (1983) Reflective learning: key to learning from experience. *Journal of Humanistic Psychology*; **23** [2]: 99–117.

Bramley P (1986) Evaluation. In: Mumford A (ed.), *Handbook of Management Development*, 2nd edn. London: Gower, pp 390–411.

Burnard P (1990) *Learning Human Skills. An Experiential Guide for Nurses*, 2nd edn. Oxford: Heineman Nursing.

Casey D (1991) The shell of your understanding. In Pedlar M (ed.), *Action Learning in Practice.* London: Gower, pp 297–305.

De Bono E (1967) *The Use of Lateral Thinking.* Harmondsworth: Penguin Books.

Department of Health (1993) *The Challenges for Nursing and Midwifery in the Twenty-first Century. The Heathrow Debate.* London: Department of Health.

Dewey J (1929) *Experience and Nature.* New York: Grave Press.

Easterby-Smith M and Burgoyne J (1991) Action learning: an evaluation. In: Pedlar M (ed.), *Action Learning in Practice*, 2nd edn. London: Gower, pp 341–348.

Garrett B (1987) Learning is the core of organisational survival: action learning is the key integrating process. *Journal of Management Development*; **6** (2), 38–44.

Garrett B (1991) The power of action learning. In: Pedlar, M (ed.), *Action Learning in Practice*, 2nd edn. London: Gower, pp 45–61.

Handy C (1991) *The Age of Unreason.* London: Business Books.

Honey P (1986) Styles of learning. In: Mumford A (ed.), *Handbook of Management Development*, 2nd edn. London: Gower, pp 111–124.

Hunt J (1979) *Managing People at Work.* London: Pan Books.

Kanter R (1990) *The Change Masters*, 4th impr. London: Unwin Paperbacks, 294.

Kolb D (1984) *Experiential Learning.* New Jersey: Prentice Hall.

Laing D (1959) *The Divided Self.* Harmondsworth: Penguin Books.

Lawlor A (1991) The components of action learning. In: Pedlar M (ed.), *Action Learning in Practice.* London: Gower, pp 247–259.

Lessem R (1991) A biography of action learning. In: Pedlar M (ed.), *Action Learning in Practice*, 2nd edn. London: Gower, pp 17–30.

Lewin K (1958) The group decision and social change. In: Maccoby E (ed.), *Readings in Social Psychology.* London: Holt Rinehart and Winston.

McClure ML, Poulin MA, Sovie MD, Wandelt MA (1983) *Magnet Hospitals: Attraction and Retention of Professional Nurses.* Kansas City: American Academy of Nursing.

McGill I and Beaty L (eds) (1993) *Action Learning. A Practitioner's Guide*, 2nd edn. London: Kogan Page, pp 17, 90.

Morgan G (1988) Quoted in McGill I and Beaty L (eds), *A Practitioner's Guide*. London: Kogan Page, pp 186–188.

Morgan G and Ramirez R (1984) Action learning: a holographic metaphor for guiding social change. *Human Relations*; **37**: 1–28.

Morris J (1986) The learning spiral. In: Mumford A (ed.), *Handbook of Management Development*, 2nd edn. London: Gower, pp 183–198.

Morse P (1991) Passed with flying colours. *The Health Service Journal*; **1** [52]: 20–22.

Neis ME and Kingdon RT (1990) *Leadership in Transition: A Practical Guide to Shared Governance*. Illinois: Nova I, viii, pp 112.

Orton, H (1981) *The Ward Learning Climate and Student Nurse Response*. London: Royal College of Nursing.

Pedlar M (1991) *Action Learning in Practice*, 2nd edn. London: Gower.

Peters TJ and Waterman RH (1982) *In Search of Excellence. Lessons from America's Best Run Companies*. London: Harper Row.

Rafferty AM (1993) *Leading Questions. A Discussion Paper on the Issues of Nurse Leadership*. London: King's Fund Centre, 3.

Revans, R 1983: *The ABC of Action Learning*. England: Chartweli-Bratt.

Rogers C (1979) *Carl Rogers on Personal Power*. London: Constable.

Schon D (1983) *The Reflective Practitioner*. London: Temple Smith.

Swieringa J and Wierdsma A (1992) *Becoming a Learning Organisation*. Cambridge: Cambridge University Press.

Toffler A (1973) *Future Shock*. England: Pan.

Tuckman BW (1965) Development sequences in small groups. *Psychological Bulletin*; **63** [6]: 384–399.

Wright S (1989) *Changing Nursing Practice*. London: Edward Arnold.

7 Nursing in a business culture. Developing a framework for total quality management

Carmel Hale and Maureen Hampson

The National Health Service reforms of the last decade have dramatically changed the clinical and business function of hospitals, (DOH, 1983, 1989a,b). This chapter demonstrates how one trust hospital met the challenge of moving into a more business orientated culture, without adversely affecting the delivery of high quality health care. The philosophy of total quality management (TQM) and the implications of this within the trust are examined. In doing this, the aim is to raise awareness of how business and quality concepts can be applied to a clinical setting and influence changes in patient care.

Total quality management

Total quality management is not a new concept within this country, but it is new to the health care market. The principles of TQM were developed by quality gurus such as Deming (1986) and Juran (1989). It originated in the United States, but flourished in Japan after World War II. It is a philosophy adaptable to all management areas, including service, industry, and education, (Rehder and Ralston, 1984). In business terms, TQM can be viewed as a cost effective system which facilitates the integration of people, services, and quality to deliver customer satisfaction. The philosophy of TQM is at present used throughout the industrial arena, and may alter the way business and management practices are conducted throughout the world (Stuelpnagel, 1989).

What is TQM and where does it fit within a hospital environment?

In answering these questions there is a need to define quality. Most people have differing views on this, because quality means different things to different people.

> Quality has a particular and simple definition in the TQM philosophy: Meeting Customers' Requirements. Under this definition, it is the customer of a product or service who defines the quality of what is delivered. The customer knows what he or she wants and only the customer can decide whether or not it is up to scratch (NHS Management Executive, 1993a).

TQM can be implemented within a manufacturing or service industry, and as Reed (1992) states, 'TQM is not a prescription for remedying flaws; it is about changing the culture of an organization, to achieve tangible benefits for both patients and staff'. Quality has become so important in the delivery of health care that it is essential that everybody within the organization has the same understanding of what quality is.

In the authors' workplace it was agreed that TQM meant 'continuously meeting agreed customer requirements at the lowest cost, by releasing the potential of all its employees' (Aintree Hospitals, 1992).

TQM within the trust

Quality was recognized by the trust as fundamental to a clear vision of the duty of the organization to provide high quality health care. It was acknowledged that quality was easy to say, but far more difficult to achieve without knowledge, understanding, and a carefully managed approach.

A working group led by the chief executive of the trust was formed to outline clearly the fundamental principles of continuous improvement, and a strategic document was prepared (Aintree Hospitals, 1991b). This document emphasized:

• High quality health care.
• Getting everyone involved.
• Making quality everyone's business.

The Nursing and Quality Director conducted a literature review of current TQM processes, and attended external events and company visits. An external management consultant was selected to assist in planning the way forward. Workshops were held for all managers from all disciplines, including consultant medical staff. Fifty-three staff employees from various disciplines received intensive training as quality facilitators. This enabled them to assist their departments in the implementation of TQM, by utilizing their specific knowledge of the tools and techniques in quality improvement.

Empowerment of staff

TQM involves all the levels of an organization, services and staff. The essence of TQM is empowerment – empowering individuals to take responsibility for improving their services/practice. As Arikian (1991) states, 'Nurses, the largest workforce within most health care organizations, must seek effective ways not only to provide high quality professionalism and service but to lead other members of the health care team in doing likewise'. All grades of staff have special skills and knowledge worth utilizing, and by giving them the opportunity and support they require, managers can maximize their enthusiasm and potential. Empowered staff are able to take responsibility for their actions, seek new ways to meet new situations, or better ways to meet the usual situations, and therefore offer a more individualized service. This empowerment decentralizes decision making and increases individual professional accountability (Pearson, 1989).

The principles of total quality management

From the outset, it was important to identify those principles of TQM that were more closely related to the trust's own philosophy. This philosophy emphasized grass roots innovations which utilize effective resource management, and also the setting of quality improvement targets. The links with TQM principles were obvious. The following list, taken from the *Aintree Hospitals TQM Facilitators' Manual* (1992–3), demonstrates this.

Managers lead by example

Managers must lead change through continuous improvement. They should agree goals, plan agendas, and communicate. Without a clear lead from the management, it would be impossible for a TQM culture to succeed. Developing a positive two-way communication process between management and staff becomes essential.

Effective communication is the key

All staff must communicate effectively. This is a three-way process:

- to the people working for you;
- to the people you work for;
- to the people you work with.

Following each month's executive trust board meeting, information is cascaded throughout all levels of the authors' organization within a defined 48-h period. This is known as team briefing.

Identify customer supplier chains

TQM has led to an emphasis on meeting the needs of the consumer through services provided by the organization. A complex network of internal and external customers now exists. External customers, that is general practitioners and purchasing authorities, buy packages of care for their patients. Customers within the organization are involved in purchasing packages of care and services to meet their patients' needs.

Agree customer requirements

Before agreeing customer requirements, it is necessary to ensure that you know who your customers are. The most efficient method of ascertaining what customer requirements are is to ask the customers. This may seem obvious, but it is all too easy for staff to assume that they know already what the customers want.

Training in quality management is essential

TQM is about meeting customers' requirements. This can only happen if staff are properly trained both in their job and in how to make and control the changes that need to happen. As Arikian (1991) states, 'training will help nurses do it right the first time, make fewer mistakes, waste less time, use fewer materials, and increase efficiency and productivity.'

Do the right things right first time

This means understanding what is required of you and making sure that you have what you need to do the job. Giving the customers what they need, getting it right the first time, is the only acceptable standard for your work.

Performance measurement is critical

Unless you can measure something, how will you know if it is right? One of the key steps is to find a way of measuring performance in actual figures. Agree your target and measure against it.

Recognize success and praise it

The recognition of success is important to staff if they are to be empowered to make further changes. Staff feel valued when they are praised for their contributions and achievements.

Continuous improvement is the goal

The fundamental point of the quality philosophy is to ensure a continuous improvement of quality in both health care and resource management. This necessitates all grades of staff being engaged in systematic and well thought out review programmes, enabling a business-like culture to develop.

Business culture and TQM

Nurses have faced unprecedented changes in recent years. These changes require them to evaluate critically all areas of their professional, managerial, and clinical practice. It is no longer acceptable that issues relating to clinical practice be seen as separate from business planning. The Audit Commission reports (1991, 1992) noted that nursing had often been left to develop in isolation from the corporate direction. This was one of the reasons why it was proposed that nurses should adopt the principles of TQM. The framework for the continuous measurement of clinical practice within a business culture is demonstrated in the trust's strategy documents (Aintree Hospitals, 1991a,b,c, 1992, 1993–4).

Mission statements

Mission statements are used within many public and non profit-making organizations. Current thinking on mission statements could be said to have originated in the 1970s; but as long ago as 1957 David Selznick (cited by Klemm et al., 1991) saw a mission statement as a means of identifying a company's distinctive competence. In 1974 Peter Drucker also focused upon the need for a business to define its purpose. There is no single satisfactory definition of what a mission statement is; but perhaps the best available is that the mission statement concerns the long term purpose of the hospital, which reflects deeply held corporate views. The mission statement of each directorate within a hospital should tie in very closely with the corporate statement. Here is an example of a directorate mission statement: 'The aim of the directorate/department is to provide quality health care to meet the needs of the individual client'. It can be seen from this what the purpose of the directorate/ department is and how it takes account of long term aims, objectives, and values.

Holt (1993) suggests that managers need to review their internal and external environments to ensure that their mission reflects the values and strategic direction of their organization. There is a need to evaluate the progress and effectiveness of a mission statement. In today's political climate, a service has to be provided that is both relevant and available to the local population.

Business planning

The creation of a business culture requires staff understanding the principles behind it. Business planning within the NHS is a comparatively new activity. Any business needs to plan in order to manage, and its planning activities are intended to enable the organization to move into a desired future position. In the past, planning activities in the NHS were centrally driven, and information was not always available when it was needed; when it was available, it was often too generalized and out of date.

The development of the NHS reforms and the introduction of greater competition has brought about major changes in the traditional roles of all NHS managers. Since April 1991 there has been a fundamental change in the NHS philosophy, with the establishment of self governing hospitals (DOH, 1989a,b). This has created a market led culture by the creation of the internal market, the recognition that there are purchasers and providers of health care, and the introduction of competition and choice.

Business planning takes place within this market, but it now relates to internal performance management which involves all nurses and clinicians in management. Each speciality – for instance surgery, medicine, or urology – has its own market. It differs from area to area, depending on the way business is conducted. Each ward/department is supplied internally with services from clinical support departments, such as pathology, radiology, pharmacy, and non-clinical support departments, such as catering, linen services, and sterile supplies.

Internal business arrangements are beginning to evolve, leading to internal customer and supplier relationships. This is the basis on which business planning begins to address the market.

Business planning should not be viewed solely as a management or corporate issue, but should indicate the effectiveness of the nursing care delivered. For this reason, nurses must be involved in the business planning process. Nurses need to demonstrate how practical issues are paramount when clinical and managerial initiatives are being considered. They need also to be aware of professional and budgetary influences.

First steps

Having considered the impact TQM and business planning have on today's NHS, it is necessary to address these issues in the context of clinical practice. The following are the stages by which the authors dealt with these issues within their own trust.

Setting up a group

Initially, a group of nurse managers within the organization was identified to highlight areas of innovative clinical practice. They developed a working framework which paid particular attention to the trust's nursing strategy (Aintree Hospitals, 1992).

The group's strategy

At the first meeting it was agreed that the group should concentrate initially on developing a framework for existing areas of practice. This would avoid the fragmentation of practice throughout the trust. Since clinical areas are faced with a continually changing environment, it was felt that the group should examine critically all aspects of their present working practices. With this in mind, it was agreed to complete a department purpose analysis in each working area. This is critical in applying the concepts and principles of TQM in a practical way, since it provides a clear focus for agreeing, measuring, and meeting customer requirements. It is designed to ensure a department or group is achieving goals, and to contribute and add value to the organization's vision, strategy, and objectives. At this point it was recognized that much of the work required was already occurring within directorates. Therefore at this stage the aim of the group was to provide a framework/model for incorporating these issues.

Examining current practice

The group decided to examine current practices by using the following framework:

- to review existing ward philosophies and ensure that they were measurable;
- to carry out the department purpose analysis (DPA);
- to prioritize any identified stressors;
- each area to develop a mission statement relating to the directorate and the corporate mission statement;
- each member of the group to select measurable objectives for each ward.

A DPA is a process of five main steps and questions (Aintree TQM Manual, 1992–3):

Step 1 Key activity statement
What do we think we do?
What skills/talents do we have?
Step 2 Purpose and goals
Does this line up with business mission/goals/priorities?
Does our manager agree?
Step 3 Customer/supplier review
Who are our customers and suppliers?
What are their requirements?
How should we measure our/their performance?
Step 4 Time and skills analysis
What do we actually do?
How do we use our time/resources?
What are the opportunities for improvement?
Step 5 Action plan
What do we need to do to make the improvements?
How do we hold onto the gains?

All of the group members felt that completing a DPA enabled them to focus on their own areas, and to identify opportunities both as immediate gains and quality improvement projects. It was seen as an opportunity to involve large numbers of managers and staff in the TQM business of the organization.

Ward philosophy

Each ward had a philosophy, but the main finding of the group was the lack of connection to the hospital's nursing strategy and directorate business plans. Nursing staff expressed difficulty in making the philosophy explicit, understandable by others, and measurable. Group members found, on reviewing their philosophies, that nursing staff incorporated all aspects of the patient's physical, social, economic, and religious needs, instead of describing the ward as it actually was and not some idealistic and unrealistic working environment. This led to the problem of measuring outcomes of care within existing ward philosophies.

The rewriting of ward philosophies was achieved when group members liaised with their own wards to address the main problem of developing a coherent structured statement of individual values and beliefs. These statements had to be realistic and pertinent to their particular speciality, and fit within the trust's nursing strategy, corporate objectives, and each directorate's business plan. This fits with the definition given by Place (1990) that 'the philosophy is not just a statement of beliefs but signifies a multidisciplinary approach to ward based health care'. A ward philosophy can be a powerful tool for change.

Developing a framework

Having successfully completed the rewriting of ward philosophies, the group was spurred on to address the other issues mentioned. At this point Lewin's (1958) work was considered to be the most appropriate framework for the facilitation of the change. The main stages of Lewin's change process are:

The unfreezing process

At this stage motivation in staff must be present to create some sort of change to occur.

The moving stage

Moving is the change itself based on information sought by staff to clarify and identify the problem. Lewin believes that looking at the problem from a different perspective gives more solutions from which to choose. It might also increase the time it takes to make a decision about the best possible solution to the problem. In this second stage the change itself is planned out and initiated.

The refreezing stage

This occurs when individuals integrate the ideas into their own value system.

Another of Lewin's theories of change is that there are driving forces and restraining forces at work, which facilitate or impede the process of change. It is important to identify these driving and restraining forces so that they can work and be capitalized on. Effective change in patient care is dependent not only on the selection of appropriate frameworks, but also on the active involvement of the participants. Haffer (1986) therefore argues that two important issues need to be considered in selecting the appropriate strategy to facilitate change: the focusing of the strategy on the appropriate change target; and the willingness and ability of the group to change.

A seven-stage framework was developed from Lewin's theory as cited by Lippitt in Welch (1979) which was found to be relevant to nursing. These seven stages are:

1. Identification of the problem

Within the profession there is an assumption that nurses understand and can apply to their clinical practice such concepts as collaborative care planning, auditing, outcome measurements, and key standard targets. The group recognized that some areas might not be meeting the basic requirements within the trust's nursing strategy, mission statement, corporative objectives, and business plan.

2. Assessment of motivation and capacity for change

The second stage, the planning stage, involved the identification of key staff to form a group that would impact at ward level. Their ideas and experiences would have to shape the process of change and develop innovative practice. The group identified nurses who had shown an interest and were committed to the development of nurse practice.

3. Assessment of the change agents, motivation, and resources

The ability of the group members to motivate staff and guide developments effectively is essential to achieve any success with innovative practices. For this reason, ward nurse managers with these skills were selected to head the project for specific directorates within the trust. They were practitioners who had a proactive and innovative approach. The group recognized that they would need support and commitment from their staff at ward level.

4. Selecting progressive change objectives

At this stage it is useful to have deadlines to work to. This helped in moving the group forward towards decision making. Therefore the group members decided to consider three main aspects from the trust's nursing strategy. These were quality, resource management, and professional development. They decided to examine working practices within individual wards and departments and identify objectives from these three aspects. It was important that each objective should be dated and have a measurable outcome, so that it could be monitored and audited. It was agreed that the group would concentrate on three main areas – professional development, resource management, and quality – and formulate objectives considering the following documents: *The Health of the Nation* (DOH, 1992); *The Patients' Charter* (DOH, 1991); the trust's corporate/directorate/ward objectives. It was agreed that in their next meeting the group would concentrate on the following three objectives and develop ways to measure and monitor them: the named nurse; professional development; health education.

5. The role of the change agent

This role was considered to be of importance as success or failure depended on individuals being able to implement change within their own environments. All the group members reported positive feedback after successfully motivating their colleagues. When they talked through the group's work with ward colleagues and asked for their assistance, most wards had taken ownership of the objectives. It was found that the wards had tackled each objective in a very similar way.

6. The maintenance of change

Group members felt that communication was vital. Frequent meetings with ward colleagues were considered essential, in order to maintain interest and keep nurses informed. Support from managers was welcomed by the group members, as this demonstrated their commitment.

7. The withdrawal of the change agent

In the final stage the change agent withdraws from the situation, leaving his or her colleagues to maintain the change alone and gradually take over the functions of the change agent.

Although Lippitt (1979) identified seven stages in the process, it is important to remember that none of these divisions is rigid, as the change process may run back and forth between the stages.

Practical application of the three objectives

This section shows how one department developed objectives in relation to the named nurse, health education, and professional development and how TQM influenced this process. Local audit tools were developed to monitor the processes: it is just as important to measure a process as it is to deliver it. What is measured should be beneficial to the individual as well as to the organization as a whole. It is intended to demonstrate how measurement can be simple, visible, and easy to calculate, and therefore understandable by all the staff. Until performance is measured, it is difficult to envisage how much scope there is for improvement.

Example 1. The named nurse

The named nurse concept is included in *The Patients' Charter* (1991) which seeks to extend consumer rights, and it is therefore everyone's business. Carr (1992) states, 'People involved in hands on delivery of patient services must own the Charter, while senior managers should face the fact that good managers live vicariously and act on behalf of the patients and staff'. The Charter highlights the need for a named qualified nurse, midwife, or health visitor to be responsible for the patient's nursing or midwifery care. In addressing this objective, the group wrote a standard which identifies three main areas: structure, process, and outcome methodology (Donabedian, 1980). This standard was then validated by the clinical quality advisor (*see* Tables 7.1 and 7.2). The monitoring tool was then developed, addressing identified issues within the structure, process, and outcome framework, and then used by the senior nurse to monitor the standard. The named nurse audit tool (Table 7.3) was developed and implemented. The results of the audit within the directorate were as follows:

10 patients were asked if they knew the name of their nurse (see Figs 7.1 and 7.2).
6 knew the full name of their identified named nurse.
4 either did not know or were unsure.

Of these four patients, two knew the first name only of their named nurse, although this was not highlighted in the results. This resulted in an 84% compliance

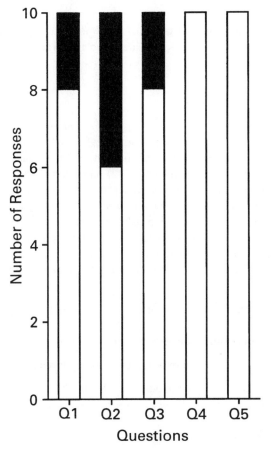

Figure 7.1   Responses to questions.
■ NO, □ YES.

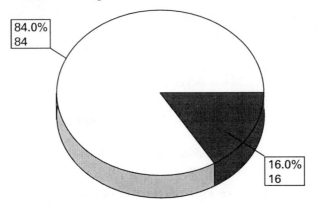

Figure 7.2   Compliance to standard ref AH/DS/010/92.
☐ Compliance, ■ Non-compliance.

rate (see Fig. 7.2) with a revised target of 100% to be attained within the next 6 months. This enabled shortcomings to be identified and an action plan developed for re-auditing in 6 months' time.

Example 2. Health education

The fundamental philosophy of *Working for Patients* (DOH, 1989a) is to add years to life and life to years, to promote health and prevent illness, and to improve diagnosis, treatment, and rehabilitation, and the quality of the environment. *The Health of the Nation* (DOH, 1992) had a major impact at ward level, with its emphasis on health promotion rather than disease prevention.

Two targets from *The Health of the Nation* (DOH, 1992) are: increasing awareness among the population of the main risk factors associated with coronary heart disease and strokes; increasing awareness among the population that it is possible to do something to reduce the personal risk of coronary heart disease and strokes. This external directive resulted in the following objectives being written by ward staff:

- health education leaflets concerning strokes are available to patients and relatives on the ward;
- each ward has an identified nurse responsible for health education.

Initially these objectives were monitored by devising three simple questions:

- Has each ward a supply of health education leaflets?
- Has each ward a nominated nurse responsible for maintaining supplies of leaflets?
- Have these been monitored monthly?

The answers showed that leaflets were not always available on wards. Initially, only one nurse on the unit was responsible for the supply of leaflets. Following the

Table 7.1   Aintree Hospitals NHS Trust – Standard Monitoring Guidelines

REF NO.............AH/DS/010/92   VALIDATION SIGNATURE...................................

TOPIC.....................Patients' Satisfaction   MANAGERS SIGNATURE ....

SUB-TOPIC...............The Named Nurse

CARE GROUP...............Medicine for the Elderly

STATEMENT ....All patients and their main carers are informed of a named nurse and other nursing team members responsible for their care.

Structure	Process	Outcome
Qualified nurse grade 'E' or above	The patients are informed on admission of the name of their named nurse and other nursing team members	All patients and/or their main carers know:
Identification card – complete with nurses' names and ward extension number	The patients/main carer is given the nurse's identification card	1 The named nurse responsible for their care
Bed name card	Bed cards are clearly visible with the patient's name and the named nurse completed	2 Other nursing team members names
Nursing	Nurses' name badges are clearly visible to all patients and carers	3 Ward extension number
Team members		

Table 7.2   Aintree Hospitals NHS Trust – Standard Monitoring Guidelines

MONITORING REQUIREMENTS

PERSONS RESPONSIBLE AH/DS/010/92

What	How	Quality improvement target	Who	Standard review date
Patient's main carers know who their named nurse is	Discharge check list with regards to the named nurse	100% of all patients and their main carers known who the patient's named nurse is	Primary nurse	bimonthly (12.11.92)
Organization of care	Ward audit		Ward manager	October 1993

Table 7.3 Aintree Hospitals NHS Trust – Standard Monitoring Guidelines

Ref No: AH/DS/010/92

Standard statement: ....All patients and their main carers are informed of a named nurse and other nursing team members responsible for their care.

Ward/Department..

Name of person completing checklist:..

Ask 10 patients each month.

Date	Month 1		Month 2		Month 3	
	Yes	No	Yes	No	Yes	No
Did a nurse introduce her/himself to you as your named nurse during your admission?						
Did you know the name of your named nurse?						
Did you receive care from your named nurse?						
Did you receive care from the same team of nurses?						
Did you know the name of any of the staff that have been caring for you?						
On the display board have you: Up to date relevant information? Staff photographs on display?						
Are all staff wearing their name badges?						
How many are not? Nurses Doctors Domestics Physiotherapists Occupational therapists						
Total number of responses						

audit, an action plan was developed and an identified nurse with a particular interest in health education was given lead responsibility for health education in their particular area/ward. The nurse then, in partnership with the patient, incorporated health education into each care plan.

Example 3. Professional development

Professional development is a wide ranging subject, and wards had many objectives concerned with this topic. For the purpose of this chapter only one example is used, the professional profile. This aimed to address some of the issues raised by *Post Registration Education and Practice Project* (UKCC, 1990, 1994) and *Vision for the Future* (DOH, 1993). The objectives involved all staff completing a professional profile to assist in their professional development, and for planned courses to be facilitated for the same purpose.

The personal professional profile provides evidence of professional knowledge and competence. Nursing is a practice based profession, and education is a tool to improve practice. The profile promotes self awareness and self development by providing a record of educational activities, career progression, and work experience.

To facilitate this, a number of 'time out' sessions were arranged. This allowed ward staff an opportunity to review their roles and identify their professional development requirements. An audit document was developed by a group of ward staff and the following questions were asked: have all members of staff completed their profiles with the ward nurse manager? It was found that only a minority of staff had attempted to develop a personal profile. When staff completed their profiles with the ward managers, it enabled the ward managers to identify specific educational needs that both complemented and promoted innovative practice.

The framework for TQM: nursing and business

Within the authors' trust this project has enabled nurses to understand the main elements of clinical practice developments and how these fit within the organization's mission statement, corporative objectives, business planning, TQM philosophy, local and national nursing strategies, and the political issues that affect the NHS.

In the new era of consumer choice, general practitioner fundholding, and purchasing authorities buying services from provider units, nurses will need to have a greater awareness of the services they offer (NHS Management Executive, 1993b). Nurses need also to understand the implications these have at ward level in the delivery of patient care. Wright (1986) supports the view that nurses need continually to review their values and practices, because of the demands made by the public on the nursing profession and by the profession on nurses. The more prepared and knowledgeable nurses are, the stronger the profession will become.

Moores (DOH, 1993) talks of the importance of involving nurses, midwives, and health visitors at a strategic and operational level in the purchasing of health care. If quality and cost effective health care are to be available to meet local needs, nursing development must form a part of the corporate strategic direction. This brings us back to the trust's emphasis on quality being the centre of its organizational development plans and on the need to embrace TQM across the whole organization.

This project has sought to draw together some of the current innovations in nursing, which can also be used as valuable information by managers to support contract negotiations with purchasing authorities. The monitoring of quality nursing care enables nurses to incorporate expected outcomes of planned care and demonstrate commitment to change based on the evaluation of how the nursing care is delivered.

Quality management in health care is not new. Since the establishment of the NHS, people working in hospitals and community settings have been striving in different ways to provide good health care and service. 'Total Quality Management ensures these efforts are harnessed, co-ordinated, and applied to all aspects of the complex and diverse services which make up today's NHS' (Aintree Hospitals, 1992).

References

Aintree Hospitals (1991a) *Mission Statement*. Unpublished.
Aintree Hospitals (1991b) *Quest for Quality. Strategy and Quality Document*. Unpublished.
Aintree Hospitals (1991c) *3 Rs Strategy*. Unpublished.
Aintree Hospitals (1992) *Nursing and Midwifery Strategy*. Unpublished.
Aintree Hospitals (1992–3) *Total Quality Management. Facilitator's Manual*. Unpublished.
Aintree Hospitals (1993–4) *Corporate Objectives*. Unpublished.
Arikian VL (1991) Total quality management. Application to nursing service. *Journal of Nursing Administration*; **21** [6]: 46–50.
Audit Commission (1991) *Virtue of Patients. Making the Best Use of Nursing Resources*. London: HMSO.
Audit Commission (1992) *Homeward Bound*. London: HMSO.
Carr S (1992) Patients rule, OK? *Health Service Journal*; **102** [5312]: 31.
Deming WE (1986) *Out of Crisis. Quality, Productivity, and Competitive Position*. Cambridge: Cambridge University Press.
Department of Health (1983) *The NHS Management Inquiry. Griffiths Report*. London: HMSO.
Department of Health (1989a) *Working for Patients. The White Paper*. London: HMSO.
Department of Health (1989b) *Working for Patients. Self-governing Hospitals' Working Paper 1*. London: HMSO.
Department of Health (1991) *The Patients' Charter*. London: HMSO.
Department of Health (1992) *The Health of the Nation. A Strategy of Health in England*. London: HMSO.
Department of Health (1993) *Vision for the Future. Nursing and Midwifery. Contribution to the Future*. London: NHS Management Executive.
Donabedian A (1980) *The Definition of Quality and Approaches to its Assessment*. Ann Arbor: Michigan Health Administration Press.
Drucker PF (1974) *Management: Tasks, Responsibilities, and Practices*. London: Harper & Row.

Haffer A (1986) Facilitating change. *Journal of Nursing Administration*; **16** [4]: 18–22.
Holt PR (1993) Beyond resource management towards total quality. *International Journal of Health Care Quality Assurance*; **6** [5]: 24.
Juran J (1989) Juran on leadership for quality. An executive handbook. In: Flarey DL (ed.), *Quality Improvement Through Date Analysis – Concept and Applications.* New York: Free Press.
Lewin K (1958) The group decision and social change. In: Maccoby E (ed.), *Readings in Social Psychology*. London: Holt Rinehart & Winston.
Lippitt R (1979) In: Welch LB, Planned change in nursing theory. *Nursing Clinics of North America*; **14** [2]: 307–321.
NHS Management Executive (1993a) *The Quality Journey.* London: NHS Management Executive, 2.
NHS Management Executive Nursing Directorate (1993b) *The Professional Nursing Contribution to Purchasing. A Study by the King's Fund College.* London: NHS ME.
Pearson A (ed.) (1989) *Primary Nursing*. London: Chapman & Hall.
Place B (1990) Write a ward philosophy. *Nursing Standard*; **4** [36]: 53.
Reed S (1992) Bear necessities. *Health Service Journal*; **102** [5316]: 26.
Rehder R and Ralston F (1984) Total quality management. A revolutionary management philosophy. *South American Adv. Management Journal*; **49** [3]: 25.
Selznick B (1957) In: Klemm N, Sanderson S, Luffman G (1991) Mission statements. Selling corporate values to employees. *Long Range Planning*; **24** [3]: 73–78.
Stuelpnagel TR (1989) TQM is business and academia cited in: Arikian VL (ed.) 1991, *Business Forum*; **14** [1]: 4–9.
United Kingdom Central Council for Nursing, Midwifery, and Health Visiting (1990) *Post Registration Education and Practice Project*. London: UKCC.
United Kingdom Central Council for Nursing, Midwifery, and Health Visiting (1994) *The Future of Professional Practice. The Council's Standards for Education and Practice Following Registration*. London: UKCC.
Wright SG (1986) *Building and Using a Model of Nursing*. London: Edward Arnold.

Appendix 1   Aintree Hospitals NHS Trust Mission Statement

Statement of commitment

Our purpose is to provide high quality health care. To this end, we are committed to:

Our patients

- by delivering effective and efficient patient care in a manner which respects people's dignity, privacy, and individuality; and
- by giving all relevant information to patients and, with their consent, to their relatives and friends on treatment progress.

Our staff

- by providing basic training, continuing education and staff development facilities and opportunities.

Our organization

- by creating an organizational climate that offers a courteous service to all users in a pleasant and compassionate environment;
- by encouraging honest and open communication and involving all staff in the planning and direction of their work; and
- by achieving effective and efficient use of our resources.

Our future

- by encouraging teaching and research in developing our acute hospitals to maintain and enhance their reputation as centres of excellence;
- by developing progressively diagnostic and treatment services for local people;
- by seeking continuous improvements in the use of new technology, developments in patient care and the amenities provided by the hospitals;
- by working in partnership with general practitioners, health and local authorities, and other providers in North Merseyside and our extended service area.

Appendix 2   Aintree Hospitals NHS Trust Corporate Objectives 1993–4

1   To manage hospital services effectively within the income received from the purchasers. This will include achieving quality performance targets and continuously improving asset utilization.

2   To implement the Aintree Hospitals Strategic Plan to relocate all hospital inpatient services on the Fazakerley site at the earliest opportunity.

3   To create an organizational climate of open management, honesty, and teamwork through a human resources strategy which recognizes these corporate values and promotes the involvement of all staff in the planning and direction of their work with a view to achieving continuous improvement in quality and productivity.

4   To continue the quality improvement programme by implementing performance management in all directorates and service departments, which will incorporate the recognition of successful achievements.

5   To improve the public image of Aintree Hospitals by implementing a communications strategy which:

- enables a two-way information flow with staff at all levels in the organization;
- recognizes the important partnership we form with general practitioners, health and local authorities and other providers in North Merseyside and our extended service areas; and
- informs the public about our efforts to improve access, quality standards and the developing range of services available within the Aintree Hospitals.

6   To develop a business plan which addresses the health needs of the local community, which aims to improve market share by identifying opportunities to expand services with clinical and other services with the relevant capacity and expertise.

7   To promote a partnership between management and clinicians which is based on common understanding of corporate aims, objectives and values in order to improve corporate performance.

8   To agree contracts with the North Mersey Health Consortium, other corporate purchasers and general practitioners, to ensure that existing and developing patient services are properly funded and progress is made in improving quality standards to meet both internal and external criteria.

9   To create a learning and innovative culture within the hospital's departments, including seeking out new opportunities for developing health care services and developing clinical/service excellence, measured by appropriate audit systems and resulting in increased patient confidence and satisfaction.

10   To develop an information culture to ensure that the trust has sufficient information to enable it to address performance management issues, using existing information, improving local information systems and ultimately implementing integrated computer systems when the benefits of such have been assessed and considered realizable.

8 When two worlds collide: nursing reflections on the relationship between complementary therapy and Western medicine in modern health care

Thomas Shea and Nicola Leather

> Science is the tool of the Western mind, and with it one can open more doors than with bare hands. It is part and parcel of our understanding, and obscures our insight only when it claims that the understanding it conveys is the only kind there is.
>
> (Jung, 1978)

The last 25 years has witnessed a steady growth in the number of people dissatisfied with the methods and approach of Western medicine. This has led to an upsurge in the popularity of therapies that offer a different ethos, manner and style to conventional, medical orthodoxy. The upper echelons of the medical profession have greeted the resurgence of complementary approaches with guarded optimism (British Medical Association, BMA, 1993). This type of response has been provoked largely because there is little empirical evidence that the beneficent outcomes of complementary intervention can be scientifically substantiated (Lancet, 1983). Other practitioners, notably nurses, have welcomed the opportunities which complementary therapies can promote with dynamism and enthusiasm (Griffin, 1993; Malkin, 1994; Pfiel, 1994).

The central thrust of this chapter is not to explore the pragmatic realities of giving complementary care but to cast a critical gaze over conceptual issues which both underpin and impinge upon its delivery. The focus and direction of this process will take the following form:

1 *The evolution of the medical model.* It is impossible to ask why medicine enjoys such a powerful position unless the themes surrounding its evolution are critically considered. This will involve an examination of the key elements involved in the development of the medical model and trace some of the factors which have influenced its position of dominance.

2 *Dissatisfaction with orthodox medicine.* The current vogue suggests a dissatisfaction with the mechanisms and delivery of orthodox medicine (Hope, 1989). The reasons behind this need to be carefully considered. What will emerge is an analysis of the influencing factors that have led increasing numbers of both lay and professional health workers to express frustration at the methods of Western orthodoxy.

3 *In medicine's shadow.* If nurses are to play a pertinent role in cultivating complementary therapies then they must develop a professional identity which is distinct from medicine. This section will explore the influence which medicine has had upon the development of nursing and make a plea for nurses to be proactive in grasping the opportunity which complementary therapies offer for expanding their role and the therapeutic options which may be offered to patients.

4 *Towards change.* There is some evidence that the dominant themes of the medical model are beginning to sway and that nurses are acting as change agents. Complementary therapies offer nurses an avenue for practice which moves beyond the restrictive confines of the medical model.

5 *Where should the buck stop?* Any innovation relating to complementary therapies and nursing needs to be examined in the light of accountability and responsibility. These themes will be considered and explored in relation to contemporary themes and complementary therapies.

6 *Above all, do no harm – avoiding negligence.* A common argument against complementary therapies is that they do not conform to the investigative pattern of the natural sciences and orthodox medicine. This section will examine the pragmatic value of terms such as 'do no harm' and ask if risk can ever be eliminated from any sort of therapeutic intervention.

The evolution of the Western medical model

The current favour with which members of the public view complementary therapies suggests a degree of dissatisfaction with the approaches of medical orthodoxy. Reflecting such themes, (Hope, 1989) suggests that people have realized that traditional Western medicine has definite boundaries: 'That is not to say that people have rejected orthodox medicine. Rather, they have recognized its limitations'. Complementary therapies offer a means of crossing new frontiers and broaden the dimensions of health care.

Despite the popularity which complementary therapies currently enjoy, traditional medicine is by far the most dominant method for delivering health care in the West. Given the influence which medicine holds, an examination of its evolution and themes will provide a degree of insight for explaining why it enjoys such a powerful position.

The main themes underpinning the development of contemporary Western medicine can be traced back to a period of history known as the Renaissance. This was a period of great intellectual growth; commenting upon the dynamism of this age, Hale (1993) states 'It saw the emergence of a new and pervasive attitude to what were considered the most valued aspects of civilized life. It witnessed the most concentrated wave of intellectual and creative energy that had yet passed over the continent'.

During this diverse and challenging period, a French philosopher named René

Déscartes rigorously questioned traditional propositions and led the way in innovative thinking. Although Déscartes contributed greatly to debates surrounding mathematical knowledge, he is also intrinsically linked to philosophical enquiry about the relationship between the mind and the body. What emerged from this was a radical treatise which confronted and challenged all convention concerning mind–body discourse.

Prior to the Renaissance, the dominant mode of thinking was that all actions were controlled and ordained by divine will. Commenting upon the manner in which Déscartes challenged such convention, Kendrick (1994) states:

> Déscartes contested these themes believing that the mind could best be seen as an autonomous entity free from external influence. Such reasoning was based on the premise that the body was directly analogous with a machine because both had parts which could break and need repair. The final stage in Déscartes' argument continued this theme and maintained that the body be studied by reducing it into components and sections. Initially, this took the form of splitting the body into systems but has progressed, with scientific advancement, to the point that we can now study at the sub-molecular level.

This philosophical perspective on the mind–body split is known as 'Cartesian Dualism'.

Déscartes' particular form of dualism has been rigorously challenged by philosophical schools in subsequent centuries, notably by the philosophical behaviourists (Ryle, 1949). Such criticisms, however, do not detract from the influence which Déscartes' thinking had in forging the cornerstone on which scientific medical enquiry was to be based. What emerged from this was the stimulus to treat parts of the body rather than the body as a whole. This provided a sharp contrast to the pre-Renaissance theme which saw the body and the mind as unified entities.

Cartesian Dualism placed the body very much under the mandate of medicine. This approach rapidly gained acceptance as the most scientifically acceptable method of discovering new knowledge about the body. Humankind has benefited greatly from this method; medical specialism has been able to offer a degree of expertise which would never have been found in the generic practitioner. As an illustration, oncology would never have existed if the pathology of cancer had not been reduced to the intricate physiology of the cell (Kendrick, 1994). Such examples give support to the main themes which underpin the medical model; if medicine's focus is upon dealing with the disease process and seeking a cure, then Déscartes' exemplar provides a firm platform for such an endeavour.

This section has given a brief overview of the main elements which contributed to the evolution of the medical model. As a mode of operation it has unrivalled success in the Western world. However, the next part of this enquiry will deal with an exploration of the possible reasons why medicine's monopoly upon the delivery of health care is being slowly challenged.

Dissatisfaction with orthodox medicine

Increased awareness of the possible benefits of complementary therapies has led people to seek further information about broader approaches to healing. Results from research carried out by Furnham and Smith (1988) revealed that people who choose complementary therapies may do so from disenchantment with, or bad experiences of, traditional medicine. Further reflecting such themes, some critics argue that orthodox medicine is actually responsible for creating illness. A seminal example of this sort of thinking is provided by the work of Illich (1976), who uses the term 'iatrogenesis' to describe the processes by which medicine causes disease. Against this backdrop, there is little wonder that interest in complementary therapies is gaining momentum.

The medical model reflects an approach towards the human condition which is value free and detached from holistic themes. Such an approach clearly builds upon Déscartes' thinking and differentiates between the mind and the body. In this respect, the mind is viewed as the realm of thoughts, feelings and emotions. It cannot be placed under a microscope or grown in a petrie dish and does not offer easy access to the traditional methodology of the natural sciences. Conversely, the physical body clearly dwells in the concrete, physical world and is open to the investigative elements and rationale of the physical sciences. Emerging from this is an approach which gives a particular view of both health and illness. Sometimes the enactment of the medical model is referred to as 'medicalization'; Ahmedzai (1993) defines this process as:

> the consequences of adopting the medical model of thinking about illness and health, which is based on an understanding (however incomplete) of pathological processes. It is assumed that as the human body is an organism, all disease states can be understood in terms of immunological, biochemical, degenerative or (increasingly) genetic malfunctions.

Describing the key elements of this method as a modus operandi, Kendrick (1992) refers to four interlinking aspects:

1 The body: the body is seen as a collection of biological systems. Each system has distinct features, but relates to the others to provide a unified whole.
2 Health: if a state of balance or homeostasis exists between the different systems in the body, then the person is said to be in a state of health.
3 Disease: disease is believed to result either from degenerative processes within the body, from chemical or physical pathogens invading the body from outside, or from a failure in one of the body's own regulatory mechanisms.
4 Treatment: once the disease process has produced measurable signs, symptoms and biochemical or physical abnormalities, then treatment begins. This is an active venture designed to halt degenerative processes, boost regulatory mechanisms or destroy the invader.

Applying the objective aspects of the medical model to individual patients allows little room for considerations of the mind or psyche. This has led some doctors to grasp the absolute themes of scientific enquiry and proclaim 'The question whether or not a person is ill, is a question of fact, not a question of feelings or personal norms' (Wulf et al., 1986).

Thinking of this sort has provoked much criticism, most of which is levelled at the pragmatic effect it can have upon patients. Reflecting such themes, Doyal and

Doyal (1984) argue that increased specialization in medicine has left knowledge and power in the hands of experts. This leaves the patient with no choice but passively to acquiesce, conform and trust in the services which are being offered. The result this has upon patients is eloquently affirmed by Doyal and Doyal in the following way:

> The mechanistic approach of medicine, its tendency to objectify human beings and its narrow focus on bodily symptoms, are often combined in the practice of an individual doctor, making the patient feel powerless, dehumanized and without resources. However, many people are now complaining about being treated as objects, and feminists in particular have formulated fundamental criticisms of both the knowledge base and the social relations involved in the production of medical care.

What is especially significant is the effect that the imposition of the medical model has had upon the development of nursing practice.

In medicine's shadow

At the start of this chapter, we affirmed that the resurgence of complementary therapies had been greeted with dynamic enthusiasm by nurses. This must, however, be viewed in the pragmatic light of the medical model's influence upon the identity and development of nursing practice. If nursing is to act as a significant conduit for the delivery of complementary therapies, it must seek to forge an identity that is distinct and free of the themes of the medical model.

There has been much talk, in recent decades, of nursing models and theoretical frameworks that are supposed to have shaped an identity which is clearly separate from the medical model. Research by Kitson (1991) would seem to throw some doubt upon the validity of such claims. In an exploration of the way that care is managed in care of the elderly environments, Kitson found that care is still organized according to tasks, routine and physical care giving; all of this being symptomatic of an approach which mirrors the influence of the medical model. Commenting upon the lack of distinction between medical and nursing frameworks, Kitson states 'When one considers the corresponding nursing care model, which could have served as the theoretical framework for the geriatric nursing care model, a major problem arises, namely that nursing does not have an operational model independent of the medical model'.

Nurses must accept some responsibility for the level of inertia which has allowed this position to continue and prosper. Again, Kitson comments upon this professional indictment by stating 'Nursing practice seemed content to follow in the wake of medical innovation and change. In consequence, nursing was unable to consider seriously the complexities involved in providing nursing care. Nursing also failed to determine its essential components and failed to build a framework that would ensure the goal of care was achieved in the practice setting'. If nursing has been reticent to establish clearly a cultural identity unique from medicine then it raises fundamental questions about the feasibility of nursing as a means of introducing complementary therapies into the professional remit.

Medicine has always been protective of its scientific base and monopoly on power; the introduction of complementary therapies confronts such themes. If nurses are to play a dynamic and formative role in giving the elements of complementary therapies cogency, force and direction then it must be done in a way that helps to forge parity in the relationship with medicine. If such themes are to rise above the rhetorical then key elements need to be established in clinical practice; central to these themes is the notion of leadership.

Towards change

There are many factors that influence the unequal relationship between medicine and nursing: biological determinism, patriarchy, class and media representations being a few examples that help to influence the whole process (MacKay, 1989, 1993; Holloway, 1992). As we have already seen, nursing has also been found wanting in respect of forming a professional identity and modus operandi which is clearly distinct from medicine. Commenting upon the influence which such themes can have upon the ethos and direction of the nursing profession, Kendrick (1994) states:

> medicine's empowerment is intrinsically linked to the disempowerment of nursing. If this situation is ever to change and autonomy become a subjective reality for practitioners then a process of enablement must take place at the 'grass roots' – nobody can ring the changes for nurses except nurses.

The current popularity of complementary therapies offers nurses a means of bringing innovation and change to the interface of practice; moreover, such developments would fit comfortably with issues surrounding the expansion of the nurse's role. What is more, when such themes are coupled to the notion of clinical leadership a dynamic can be created which presents an optimistic picture for the future of professional equity between doctors and nurses. Reflecting these themes, Holmes (1991) states:

> clinical leaders will create an environment in which therapeutic relationships with patients and collaborative relationships with other health professionals are possible. Effective application of the skills of leadership, therefore, expands the role of nurses, setting a standard for professional practice and helping to guide its development. This can only be of benefit to patients and to the quality of care they receive.

Many nurses are already acting as change agents in relation to introducing complementary therapies to their work (Mantle, 1992). Indeed, such is the level of interest being expressed by both lay and professional health care workers that centres are starting to evolve which cater solely for the delivery of complementary health care. Reflecting this trend, Faulkner (1990) highlights the work of the Wirral Holistic Centre in Merseyside which provides complementary therapies free to patients with cancer. Commenting upon the increasing numbers of patients demanding this sort of therapeutic intervention, Denton (1992) states 'What is certain is that people we care for are more and more loudly clamouring for the opportunity to receive a range of therapeutic skills from nurses'.

Developments of this nature suggest that an ideological shift is occurring in nursing. Emerging from this is a movement away from practising nursing within the restrictive confines of the medical model. Such themes are reflected by Lynch (1993), who argues that traditional mechanisms of monopoly, patriarchy and power are being challenged and moved: 'The old hierarchy, in which power was centred in a few, is giving way to an organisational network with shared power. ... Empowerment occurs as all within the network share the same vision, pool their energy and creativity, and move towards the same goal in a way that is effective and meaningful'. Such language is certainly stirring and may indeed reflect a changing shift in the contemporary culture which underpins health care. These developments, however, need analysing in relation to notions of accountability and responsibility in nursing.

'Where should the buck stop'

Nurses have always been expected to place great emphasis upon delivering excellence in practice. However, recent years has seen nursing become increasingly charged by the language of professionalism – accountability and responsibility are key tenets in this process. Considerable confusion surrounds the two terms and they are often used interchangeably.

In trying to reflect the essence of the terms, Pearson and Vaughan (1986) differentiate between them in the following way:

> While the two ideas are inextricably linked, there is a clear difference between them. Accountability implies that a situation has been assessed, a plan been made and carried out, and the results evaluated. Responsibility refers to the task or 'charge'. Thus nurses can be offered the 'charge' or responsibility for carrying out a particular action. In agreeing to accept the responsibility for that action, they become accountable for fulfilling it.

Building upon such themes, Burnard and Chapman (1993) argue that it is facile to say that a nurse is accountable for an action unless it is linked to a level of commensurate authority. Applying this to qualified practitioners, it is of little value to say that a staff nurse is both accountable and responsible for actions if this does not carry with it the level of authority needed to ensure that the action is carried out. Emerging from this, accountability can be said to reflect a willingness to be answerable for your own actions or omissions; likewise, responsibility means accepting the consequences for your own actions or omissions. When coupled to the professional setting such notions demand that practitioners are answerable for their professional activities; Kendrick (1992) gives the following example to illustrate this point:

> If you are given and accept the task of helping a patient/client with restricted mobility to exercise, then you are responsible for implementing and completing the task. At the same time, you become answerable to the client and other ruling bodies which safeguard, maintain and oversee standards of care. If the client were to fall while exercising, you might have to answer to your employers – you would attempt to show that despite the client's fall, you carried out your responsibility competently and carefully.

Notions of accountability and responsibility have to play a central part in any discussions concerning the developing role of complementary therapies in nursing practice. If we do not seek a formal process for validating the pragmatic application of such themes then the sceptical power base of orthodox medicine may remain rigid. Reflecting such notions, Sims (1988) states:

> Complementary care has aroused significant interest among nurses, who have addressed its implications for nursing at a number of international conferences. Nurses have been slow, however, to evaluate specific techniques for the potential benefits they have for patients. It may well be that the scepticism of medical colleagues has hindered this process. Personal experience attests to the difficulties in obtaining medical support for therapies such as slow stroke back massage, which may be perceived as 'bizarre' or 'way out'.

Reflecting these themes further, Pfeil (1994) argues 'While for many nurses the value of holistic approaches to health care and the need for complementary treatments are beyond doubt, most doctors are still seeking more hard evidence of the benefits of complementary therapies'.

Professional edicts clearly illustrate who the nurse is primarily accountable to: 'Each registered nurse, midwife and health visitor shall act, at all times in such a manner as to justify public trust and confidence, to uphold and enhance the good standing of the profession, to serve the interests of society, and above all to safeguard the interests of individual patients and clients' (UKCC, 1992).

The UKCC's Code of Conduct provides a series of guidelines intended to give practitioners direction on those themes which should inform accountable and responsible practice. Although the clauses within the code are not laws they do have a clear link with the tenets of common law. Building upon these legal themes, Dimond (1990) states '. . . a duty of care can be said to exist if one can see that one's actions are reasonably likely to cause harm to another person'. Such insights hold particular resonance for the application of complementary therapies by nurses.

'Above all, do no harm' – avoiding negligence

The duty of care is a component of the law of negligence which is involved with civil law, or more precisely, the law of tort which refers to wrong doing. Negligence relates to that conduct which falls below the standard established by the law for the protection of others against risk or harm. A key issue emerges here – what is a reasonable standard? In law this refers to the standard which could be reasonably expected of a man in the street. In relation to professional negligence, it refers to a person with a special skill and was established in the case of Bolam v Friern Hospital Management Committee (1957). Commenting upon this case, Brazier (1987) cites the words of Judge McNair which set precedent on what should constitute the test of a professional standard of care:

The test is the standard of the ordinary skilled man exercising and professing to have that special skill. A man need not possess the highest expert skill; it is well established law that it is sufficient if he exercises the ordinary skill of an ordinary competent man exercising that particular art.

The law relating to negligence applies to all dealings which involves a nurse caring for a patient. It is only in recent times, however, that nurses have developed a creeping awareness of the impact of the law on every aspect of daily work. Emerging from this are three key areas which each practitioner should reflect upon in relation to the implementation of complementary therapies:

1 That the ethos and themes of the UKCC's Code of Professional Conduct apply; thus, practitioners are responsible and accountable for their actions in the delivery of complementary therapies.
2 A duty of care is owed to the patient. This means that the risk of any harm should be reduced as much as possible. Such themes need to be addressed in the light of pragmatism. It would be impossible to eliminate harm from health care; for example, the very act of giving an intramuscular injection causes harm but is usually justified by the therapeutic worth of the intervention. The key word here is justification; any harm caused must be far outweighed by the beneficial outcomes. Building upon this, certain forms of massage may be a little 'rough' but this is justified by the resultant feeling of well-being.
3 In terms of negligence, practitioners should always ensure that their actions bear the signature of proficiency that the average person is expected to have in applying a particular complementary skill.

All of the previous areas are intrinsically concerned with the notion of competency. Clause three of the UKCC code of conduct asks practitioners to 'maintain and improve your professional knowledge and competence'. These themes are further reinforced by clause four, which advises practitioners to 'acknowledge any limitations in your knowledge and competence, and decline any duties or responsibilities unless able to perform them in a safe and skilled manner'. Such mandates suggest that nurses should be knowledgeable of the theoretical elements underpinning any complementary therapy and able to offer and deliver it to clients with confidence. This throws down a gauntlet to any nurse who wants to use complementary approaches in the delivery of care. If such an undertaking is not developed from an informed knowledge base and a competent skill's itinerary then the care that is offered to the client may be compromised and, ultimately, harmful.

Avoiding collision

This chapter has explored the complex themes which have allowed medicine to achieve such an elevated position of power and ascendancy in the West. What has emerged is that medicine offers a competent and valuable tool for applying scientific rationale to the body. This, however, limits the human condition to a pathological equation. Complementary therapies, when administered from a competent and responsible base, offer health care a means of viewing illness which need not be trapped within the enclaves of orthodoxy. This is not a plea for anything to be taken away from the methods and approach of Western medicine.

The essence of this chapter asks nurses to cast a critical and enquiring gaze at complementary therapies and enquire if anything can be taken which will improve the nature and method of care giving. The worlds of orthodox medicine and complementary therapies need not collide; each has much to offer and learn from the other – nurses hold a tenable position for helping to bring the two domains together.

References

Ahmedzai S (1993) The medicalisation of dying. In: Clark D (ed.), *The Future for Palliative Care: Issues of Policy and Practice*. Buckingham: Open University Press.

Brazier M (1987) *Medicine, Patients and the Laws*. Harmondsworth: Penguin.

British Medical Association (1993) *Complementary Medicine: New Approaches to Good Practice*. Oxford: Oxford University Press.

Burnard P, Chapman C (1993) *Professional and Ethical Issues in Nursing*. Harrow: Scutari Press.

Denton P (1992) Make your voice heard. *Nursing Standard*; **6** [50]: 49–51.

Dimond B (1990) *Legal Aspects of Nursing*. Hertfordshire: Prentice-Hall International.

Doyal L, Doyal L (1984) Western medicine: a philosophical and political prognosis. In: Birke L, Silvertown J (eds), *More Than Parts: Biology and Politics*. London: Pluto Press, Ch 5.

Faulkner A (1990) Autogenics neighbourhood venture. *Nursing Times*; **86** [16]: 50–52.

Furnham A and Smith C (1988) Choosing alternative medicine: a comparison of the beliefs of patients visiting a general practitioner and a homeopath. *Social Science and Medicine*; **26** [7]: 213–230.

Griffin A (1993) Holism in nursing: its meaning and value. *British Journal of Nursing*; **2** [6]: 310–312.

Hale J (1993) *The Civilisation of Europe in the Renaissance*. London: Harper Collins.

Holloway J (1992) The media representation of the nurse: the implications for nursing. In: Soothill K, Henry IC, Kendrick KD (eds), *Themes and Perspectives in Nursing*. London: Chapman & Hall.

Holmes S (1991) Clinical leadership: a role for the advanced practitioner. *Journal of Advances in Health and Nursing Care*. **1**[3]: 18.

Hope M (1989) *The Psychology of Healing*. Shaftesbury: Element Books.

Illich I (1976) *Medical Nemesis*. London: Calder and Boyars.

Jung CG (1978) *Psychology and the East*. London: Routledge.

Kendrick KD (1992) *Accountability in Practice and Research Based Care*. Didsbury: Open College Press.

Kendrick K (1994) Nurses and doctors: a problem of partnership. In: Soothill K, MacKay L, Webb C (eds), *Working Together? Interprofessional Relationships in Health Care*. London: Edward Arnold (in press).

Kitson A (1991) *Therapeutic Nursing and the Hospitalized Elderly*. Harrow: Scutari Press.

Lancet (1983) Editorial. Alternative medicine is no alternative. October 1: 773–774.

Lynch E (1993) Organisational networking: empowerment through politics. In: Marriner-Tomey A (ed.), *Transformational Leadership in Nursing*. Chicago: Mosby Year Book.

Mackay L (1989) *Nursing a Problem*. Milton Keynes: Open University Press.

Mackay L (1993) *Conflicts in Care: Medicine and Nursing*. London: Chapman & Hall.

Malkin K (1992) Use of massage in clinical practice. *British Journal of Nursing*; **3** [6]: 292–294.

Mantle F (1992) Complementary care. *Nursing Times*; **88** [18]: 43–45.

Pearson A, Vaughan B (1986) *Nursing Models for Practice*. London: Heinemann.

Pfiel M (1994) Role of nurses in promoting complementary therapies. *British Journal of Nursing*; **3** [5]: 217–219.

Ryle G (1949) *The Concept of the Mind*. London: Hutchinson.

Sims S (1988) Complementary therapies as nursing interventions. In: Wilson-Barnett J, Raiman J (eds), *Nursing Issues and Research in Terminal Care*. Chichester: John Wiley.

United Kingdom Central Council for Nursing, Midwifery and Health Visiting. (1992) *Code of Professional Conduct*. London: UKCC.

Wulf HR, Pedersen SA, Rosenberg R (1986) *Philosophy of Medicine: an Introduction*. Oxford: Blackwell Scientific Publications.

Section III

Change and Implementation
in Practice

For change to be accomplished successfully, there must be commitment and an understanding of the processes of change. Yet all too often the innovator is viewed, initially at least, with scepticism and even fear. Nevertheless, if these difficulties can be overcome, and change is harnessed, owned, and thoroughly planned, it is a powerful tool for development.

Section III of this book highlights the power of the nurse/patient relationship in the implementation of new practice. It offers a selection of strategies for the development of practice, which are drawn from the theory of nursing and also from each individual author's experience.

Each chapter is complementary to every other, in that the themes of quality, patient need and empowerment, practical application, and the celebration of nursing practice are explored in all of them.

Richards, in her chapter on the role of the health care assistant and its implications for the registered nurse, offers a comprehensive overview of the history of nursing roles. She asks and answers many challenging questions about the future of nurses and nursing. She uses examples from her own experience as a way of encouraging the reader to consider the future of nursing roles, and the pragmatism of her approach looks forward to the challenges of the twenty-first century.

Quality, a constant theme throughout the book, is evident throughout Keen and Weir's exploration of the role of the ward manager in the area of mental health. They facilitate a perception of primary nursing that is both refreshing and energizing. This provides reflections about the experience of implementing primary nursing, exploring the processes which staff and patients go through during this major change in the delivery of care, and giving the reader an insight into the practical steps involved and the rationale behind them. Once again, theory and practice go hand in hand.

Nursing is a profession which is always striving to connect its theory and its practice. Brash, McKenna and Kendrick, in their chapter on death and grieving, present a powerfully moving series of case studies of caring for dying patients from their own experiences. They encourage readers to look inside themselves and to question the accuracy of their own understanding of death and grieving. Then they related this to the care of the dying patient and the patient's family. So we are provided with a tool box of information and practical application that must enhance both thought and practice in this difficult area.

Now we move from death to birth. In her chapter on engendering excellence in midwifery care, Richardson analyses critically the changing face of midwifery. The mother and her child are of course at the centre of our concerns here. The author suggests the means for a comprehensive application of good practice in the area of midwifery.

Empowerment and informed choice are the essence of Dean's chapter on the implementation of self-medication within the setting of a ward. In order to give the reader a clear understanding of the complex processes involved, and to suggest strategies which may be employed at all the stages in the implementation of self-medication, she presents us with a fascinating series of patient–nurse dialogues.

From all of these chapters the reader can see how much commitment, energy, vision and sheer staying power are needed if nurses are to cope with, and facilitate, the necessary changes in the practice setting. It follows of course that changes will only be successful if all the members of a nursing team take their share of responsibility for them, and if they are backed up and encouraged by their leader. The picture presented in this section of the book – where theory illuminates them – must encourage us to challenge old practices and look to new ones in a spirit of enthusiasm.

The Editors
1994

9 Two levels of care – the emergence of the health care assistant and the implications for registered nurses

Janet Richards

Introduction

Nursing is functioning in an atmosphere of great change. Over the past decade, the way in which nursing has been organized and managed has altered dramatically. Primary nursing has emerged as the panacea for all ills. The nursing process and nursing models have altered the way in which patients are assessed and in which care is planned and evaluated.

Within the milieu of change, this chapter will examine the emerging health care assistant role by focusing upon the following remits:

- History of enrolled and auxillary nurses.
- Traditional role of auxillary nurses.
- Importance of training health care assistants.
- Impact of health care assistants on the role of registered nurses.

It is not the author's intention to appear to be in favour of or against National Vocational Qualifications. Hughes (1992) suggests that although nurses will be most affected by the introduction of health care assistants, they are the group who seem to have little knowledge of the subject. Therefore the aim of this chapter is to highlight and explore all the issues involved in the change that is occurring in the Health Service. Readers will then be able to draw their own conclusions as to whether or not it is a positive move forward.

Draper (1990) suggests that since the inception of the nursing process in the mid-1970s, new ideas have appeared at an alarming rate and the last two decades of nursing history have been a 'story of change'.

National Health Service Trusts have been introduced and are evolving to radically change hospital organizations. Other innovations are documented comprehensively elsewhere in this book. During a time of great upheaval nurses are striving to provide excellence in nursing practice and a caring, professional environment for their patients.

Sometimes it seems that there is a new initiative to cope with almost daily. During the last 4 years within a District General Hospital in the North West, a dynamic change has been the introduction of the health care assistant and the National Vocational Training programme. The National Council for Vocational

Qualifications (NCVQ) was set up in 1986. It followed a Governmental review of vocational training. The aim of the Council is to develop a framework of vocational qualifications for England, Northern Ireland and Wales from the planning stages, through to evaluation of the courses. In Scotland the Scottish Vocational Education Council (Scotvec) undertakes a similar role.

The philosophy underpinning the National Vocational Qualifications is the recognition of an individual's ability to show that they are competent in a particular set of tasks. The candidate is assessed in the workplace by an assessor who has been prepared and trained for this role. The qualifications awarded are recognized nationally and fit into a framework which, at present, consists of five levels.

- Level one is defined as the basic level. This award is given to those who are able to achieve minimum employment standards and work under supervision.
- Level two is the standard level: a person gaining such a grade should be able to work with minimum guidance and support.
- Level three is an advanced level. At this stage work includes more complex, skilled tasks. It is also said to be an indication of junior management roles. In the Health Service it will be included as entry criteria into nurse training.
- Level four is termed the higher level. This award is intended for management and professional occupations. This level indicates the ability to carry out work requiring higher skills such as planning and design in industry.
- Level five includes the capability to exercise personal autonomy and responsibility for others work. This might include such areas as resource allocation, 'planning, execution and evaluation' (NCVQ, 1991).

It is important to note that the United Kingdom Central Council (1986) believes that registered nurses should not be included at any level lower than five. However, it is impossible for professional bodies to dictate the level at which they can be included in the framework.

The introduction of National Vocational Qualifications into the Health Service has challenged registered nurses to look at their role and the effect health care assistants will have on their professional practice. To understand the changes brought about by the introduction of this new type of assistant it is important to reflect upon the historical events which have led to the implementation of this training scheme and the introduction of this new grade of assistant.

Where have we come from? An historical overview

In 1986, the United Kingdom Central Council for Nursing, Midwifery and Health Visiting (UKCC) published its document '*Project 2000: A New Preparation for Practice*' (1986). This proposed wide ranging changes to nursing. It said a great deal about the UKCC's perceptions of nursing and the health care needs of the British public. The Project 2000 document, envisaged a 'new practitioner' who should be a 'knowledgeable doer' and one level Registration instead of the

Register and Roll. In addition to this, the Council considered a new grade of helper who initially might be called an 'aide.' This title was abandoned by April 1987 and health care assistant has been accepted into the every day language of most nurses.

Because the UKCC envisaged just one level of Registration for trained nurses, they argued that there had to be a group of helpers who also received a training, but were not registered practitioners. The UKCC (1986) pointed out that ideally most people would want all care given by registered nurses but that it was clear that this was never going to be possible. Therefore, it was necessary to develop the role of a 'helper' (UKCC, 1986) who would work under the direct supervision of a registered nurse. The nurse would then be responsible for care given by the helper and would have to be aware of limitations in the delivery of care by that person. The UKCC received many comments about the proposed changes and particularly what was believed to be the abolition of the enrolled nurse. The UKCC (1986) made it clear, however, that although the training was to cease, there was a need to safeguard the employment of existing enrolled nurses. The Council suggested the development of more conversion opportunities for enrolled nurses and the evolution of different roles for those nurses who did not want to convert.

In many areas of the country, training for the Roll continued for some time after the Project 2000 proposals had been made. Since then, there has been a move to convert enrolled nurses to registered nurses by courses of varying length and content.

The development of enrolled nursing evolved out of the need for a second way of entry into nursing. In 1905, a Select Committe on Registration recommended that a second register be introduced for nurses who would take a shorter training and have a qualification distinct from state registered nurses (Abel-Smith, 1960). The Select Committee suggested this because it felt that there would be a lack of entrants to nursing who would be willing to undertake the 3-year training.

This move was opposed by the nursing profession. Mrs. Bedford Fenwick led the resistance to the second register. She and her supporters in the Royal British Nurses Association and the British College of Nurses believed that it was undesirable that anyone other than those who had taken the 3-year training programme should be allowed to call themselves 'nurse'.

However, the debate continued in the years following the admission of the first nurses to the Register.

During the First World War and the following decade there continued to be a great shortage of registered nurses. Many hospitals were staffed by a large number of untrained assistants working initially in Britain and then abroad. These Voluntary Aid Detachments (VADS) had been largely drawn from the upper middle classes. Their role was to work as ancillary staff to give support to qualified nurses. Many nursing leaders, including Mrs Bedford Fenwick, believed that it was wrong for untrained workers to be caring for the sick. McGann (1992) suggests that trained nurses felt that the VADs were attempting to gain formal recognition of their hospital work.

By the early 1930s there were 15 000 unqualified assistants, which rose to over 21 000 by the end of the decade (Abel-Smith, 1960).

The Athlone Committee was set up, in response to the moves by County Councils who started courses for assistant nurses employed by voluntary hospitals. In 1937, due to pressure from the British Medical Association and the College of Nursing, the Athlone Committee recommended a Roll rather than Register should be set up to enroll nurses who did not have the educational requirements to carry out the 3-year training programme. In 1939, the General Nursing Council recognized the necessity for a second grade of nurse although there was much discussion about the title that these 'nurses' should use (Abel-Smith, 1960).

By the outbreak of the Second World War, there was a gross shortage of entrants to training and a shortage of personnel in hospitals to care for the sick. Bingham (1979) writes of the large numbers of trained nurses who were posted overseas to nurse the sick and wounded.

The Horder Report made many recommendations, culminating in 1943 with the Nurses Act, which formally set up the Roll allowing for enrollment of nurses with 2 years' training.

It was thought that this move would lead to an ample supply of staff to care for the sick. However, this was not the case and in 1943 there was a drive by the Ministry of Labour to enlist the services of more auxiliary nurses. The role of the auxiliary nurse had developed from the hospital orderly who had taken on a largely domestic role.

Many auxiliary nurses were recruited and became invaluable to the hospitals at this time. Moreover, auxiliaries often preferred employment in that capacity, rather than undertaking the nurse training, as the pay was very low both for student and pupil nurses. White (1985) points out that most of the auxiliary nurses were married women who were not able to leave their homes and families to take on the extra work that training entailed. Some auxiliary nurses were actually given the qualification of enrolled nurse if they were deemed to be suitable by their employers, a practice which continued for a number of years.

From the inception of the National Health Service in 1948, the numbers of auxiliary nurses increased steadily. Dingwall et al. (1988) report that by the end of the 1950s there were 50% fewer enrolled nurses than auxiliary nurses in hospital settings.

The traditional role of the auxiliary nurse

A third grade of staff evolved and the auxiliary nurse became an integral part of the staffing of most wards and departments, in a wide variety of health care settings. It was intended that the auxiliary nurse would work under the direct supervision of trained staff, but they became a group of staff who worked on their own. They tended to perform tasks based on patient's physical needs, together with housekeeping duties. Auxiliaries often helped junior student and pupil nurses become acclimatized to the ward. Many trained nurses remember with gratitude and affection the auxiliary nurse who took them 'under her wing' on the first day of clinical experience because they were too nervous to speak to staff nurses! Buckley (1987) studied student nurses' experiences of caring for dying patients. The research found student nurses felt that they received more support and practical help in dealing with these patients from auxiliaries than trained nurses. In reality, this very important part of the National Health Service workforce actually received minimal training. The preparation for their work often amounted to little more than a brief orientation to the hospital and its routines, together with some spasmodic in-service training.

It could be argued that nurses have traditionally carried out the work that is inherently the 'female role' – that of care giving. Draper (1990) puts forward the view that historically it has been seen as a 'lay activity' undertaken by females. Bingham (1979) reminds us that nursing has always been considered the woman's role.

Auxiliary nurses performed that traditional role and until recently, many were married women with families who recieved little training for their work. It provided them with an opportunity to work in the health care system without the commitment of training or the responsibility of being a qualified nurse.

It should also be remembered that there has, and still is, a large number of untrained carers in the community caring proficiently for their chronically sick relatives. It follows, then, that there is an important role for the auxiliary nurse within the hospital environment.

Traditionally, ward routines were based around the division of tasks. The Ward Sister would allocate work and patient care to staff depending on their status and abilities. One trained nurse might be given the temperatures, pulses and blood pressures to record, another nurse allocated dressings and Sister would administer the drugs for all patients on the ward. This task allocation approach taken in nursing in the past led to auxiliaries performing jobs, which as well as being repetitive, were usually more physically demanding. Draper (1990) suggests that in task allocation nurses were unable to gain 'an integrated view of the nursing function'. It meant that auxiliaries carried out work such as tidying, replenishing stocks, giving out meals and toileting for patients. Rowden (1992) states that in the past auxiliary nurses have been 'used and abused'. There were few opportunities for auxiliary nurses to progress and 'power' in the ward was held by the trained staff. Draper (1990) argues that in striving for a professional status for nursing, trained staff have exerted the same type of power over auxiliaries as has been seen historically in the doctor–nurse relationship. Heenan (1990) discusses an anonymous article in the *Lancet* published in the same year that described doctors as dominant and in charge. Nurses were seen by the article's author to be 'subordinate, subservient and often submissive'. This type of power could be seen to be replicated in the relationship between auxiliary and registered nurses.

From this brief historical overview, it is possible to see why the role of the state enrolled nurse and its demise is linked with the emergence of the new health care assistant. Allan, cited in Fardell (1989), points out that part of the rationale for introducing one level of registered practitioner was enrolled nurses having been expected to take on roles for which they have not been trained.

Before the Registration Act of 1919, there was a move by some sections of the profession to have one grade of qualified nurse caring for the needs of the population. Their quest for one tier of staff is well documented in many nursing histories. Project 2000 has attempted, once again, to create one grade of trained staff assisted by untrained helpers. However, it has never been possible to have only one grade of nurse due to social and economic pressures. Meanwhile, demographic changes have led to a shortage in student nurses entering the profession; and financial constraints have led to an increase in the number of untrained staff. Certainly, in recent times it has become evident that nurses are an expensive commodity and it is cheaper to employ health care assistants who are trained to fulfil specific functions. It is clear, therefore, that the Health Service will never be staffed completely by qualified nurses.

Barrett (1994) questions whether or not nurses can continue to carry out their traditional roles, such as bed making, washing and feeding patients. These areas, which could be termed basic care, may be assigned to health care assistants under the direct supervision of trained nurses.

The health care assistant role is emerging and registered nurses need to be aware of the effects it will have on their practice.

The importance of training for auxiliary nurses

There has long been a need for formalized training for auxiliary nurses and recognition for the work they do within the nursing team. Their role has been abused countrywide. Certain auxiliaries have been allowed to practise greater skills than others, simply because the nurse supervising them has believed them competent to do that particular task. Rowden (1992) points out work deemed suitable for auxiliary nurses has often covered what most would see as the responsibility of a trained nurse, for example blood pressure recording, administering medications and giving suppositories. There are instances where staffing levels have resulted in a student nurse and two auxiliaries being left to care for a ward of patients at night with a night sister supervising several wards. Certain auxiliaries have been allowed to carry out dressings, while others did nothing other than the most basic of tasks such as cleaning, restocking shelves and assisting patients to the toilet. In response to the need for structured training and a standardization of the role, the introduction of the health care assistant and the National Vocational Qualifications have emerged and developed.

What is evident from this historical review is that outside influences such as socio-economic policies and political pressures have shaped the structure of nursing as we have come to know it. It is important that we become accustomed to this new grade of health care assistants. Registered nurses must be the group that determines how the role evolves and to what extent it erodes into our professional autonomy. Hughes (1992) supports this by proposing that if NVQs are tailored to meet the requirements of the service, then it is vital that nurses are involved in the development of the competencies and their assessment. Rowden (1992) believes that if nurses are unhappy with the content of National Vocational Qualifications, it is the responsibility of the profession, as the lead bodies have always welcomed nursing's input into the training standards.

The present – where have these changes led us?

In many areas of the country, existing auxiliary nurses have been trained to the National Vocational Qualification standards (NVQs). As mentioned earlier, the National Council for Vocational Qualifications' (NCVQ) function was to develop a framework to standardize existing vocational awards. This applies to all areas of industry, commerce and businesses as well as in the care sector.

Qualifications would be awarded a grade between levels one to five. Where there were no vocational qualifications such as within the National Health Service, the NCVQ worked with Lead Bodies such as the Care Sector Consortium (CSC) regarding qualifications to be awarded within the framework. In addition, the National Health Service Training Authority plays a central role in this Lead Body.

The National Vocational Qualifications are, in essence, a training to prepare an individual for a particular job rather than an education to allow someone to practice and Rowden (1992) supports this view.

At level one, the competencies to be assessed cover such activities as taking the patient to the toilet and helping the patient fulfil their hygiene needs. At this level the work is routine, similar to those areas of 'basic' care as explored earlier in the chapter.

At level two, the tasks to be assessed are more complex in nature, for example, caring for the needs of the dying patient.

Level three is, at the present, in its earliest stages but it is envisaged that such areas of care as taking and recording of blood pressures and wound dressings will be included.

National Vocational Qualifications have been widely accepted within the health care sector and assess the competence of health care assistants to carry out clearly defined skills. Training is based in the workplace although there are some theoretical based classroom sessions.

Change has been rapid and some may find it difficult to comprehend in association with many other changes which have occurred in nursing. Having seen the move away from two levels of qualified staff, it would be a great pity if the nursing profession were guilty of recreating history by again having an even more complicated hierarchical structure. A scenario could develop where a team structure might consist of the following:

- health care assistants at one of three levels of National Vocational Qualifications;
- registered general nurses with the traditional training;
- registered nurses with Project 2000 diplomas and degrees;
- registered general nurses with postgraduate degrees.

This will lead to even more confusion than when teams consisted of auxiliary nurses, state registered nurses and state enrolled nurses.

Davies, cited in Laurent (1989), does not believe health care assistants will replace the enrolled nurse or duplicate that of a professional nurse. He continues by stating that the health care assistant's function is to provide support to the professional nurse.

Resulting benefits of health care assistant training

So what are the advantages of the new health care assistant grade and what can they contribute to the patient care?

1. Training will be of positive benefit

As has already been discussed, auxiliary nurses have been contributing to care for years without any formal recognition. Therefore, it is right that they are now going to benefit from training. Auxiliary nurses are being given the opportunity to gain their National Vocational Qualifications before new entrants recruited within the National Health Service. The National Vocational Qualifications have provided a flexible system of workplace based training which has allowed for ongoing learning and assessment.

2. A diverse range of life experience has been introduced

The training schemes have encouraged people to join the National Health Service who would not necessarily have thought about becoming an auxiliary nurse. They bring to the service a range of experience which certainly makes life interesting. It has provided the opportunity for many previously unemployed people to obtain a training which has become very important to them. Initially, they were training for a period of time, after which they were not guaranteed permanent employment. However, many have now been given the opportunity of employment both in the Health Service and private sector and are continuing their training on that basis. Their previous experience has ranged from service in the Armed Forces to clerical work with communication companies. Johnston (1989) describes the new support worker as likely to be female, unemployed for many years, a housewife and in the age range of 35–55. Davies, cited in Laurent (1989) points out that one of the underlying principles of the training programme is to widen the sphere from which health care assistants are taken. This, she believes, will attract ethnic groups as well as men into the programme.

3. Training is intended to facilitate learning at a pace appropriate to the candidate

Another of the underlying principles of National Vocational Qualifications is to allow people to train at whatever speed they feel comfortable. In practice, there have to be some constraints on the time taken for the training period. This has led to some feeling pressured into completing assessments before they were ready to do so. It has also resulted in a certain amount of resentment, as the 'traditional' auxiliaries who have been assessed to NVQ level two standards believe that it has taken them years to develop the interpersonal skills necessary to do the job proficiently. They then see that there are relatively new entrants to the National Health Service who have already reached the same level in the National Vocational Qualifications because they have been assessed as competent to fulfil the criteria laid down in the standards. Some existing staff, with whom the author has come into contact, felt that they had to take part in the NVQ training scheme because, if they did not, they would be 'left behind' or passed over when job opportunities arose. It is interesting to reflect on the similarities between that group of staff and the reasons often given by trained staff for undertaking degree and diploma courses!

4. Training health care assistants will increase motivation

In the past, some auxiliary nurses have felt confused about their role and the tasks that they were allowed to carry out outside their sphere of responsibility. This sometimes led to a decrease in motivation and many cited health care assistant training as a catalyst which would improve staff morale. Robinson and Stillwell (1990) found that after the health care assistant role was introduced in one health region, staff motivation improved and resulted in a lower turnover of staff. An improvement in staff morale, it could be argued, would result in improved job satisfaction, retention of staff, and lower sickness and absence rates. A recent Royal College of Nursing Survey (Seccombe and Buchan, 1993) carried out in conjunction with the Institute of Manpower Studies, looked at the economic costs of absence from work within the NHS. It found that qualified nurses had an average of 13.8 days off due to sickness per year. Unqualified staff on the other hand were away from work due to sickness for an average of 17.3 days per year, a difference of 25%. It could be argued that training raises people's expectations of what their job entails and what their new role will be. If they then find that the job is not what they envisaged it to be they may become demotivated and sickness and absenteeism could rise. This could particularly apply to the auxiliaries who undertake the training and feel that, despite a great deal of hard work, their role has not altered. Adversely, it could be argued as Robinson and Stillwell (1990) found, that training increases staff morale and gives them a greater degree of professional awareness and so they are less likely to be away from work through sickness and absence.

5. Financial implications

There are important financial implications for the National Health Service when considering the emotive subject of skill mix.

Attempts to look at alternative ward and department staffing structures have been met with dismay by many nurses. Gibbs et al. (1991) describes the 'strong passions aroused by the debate'. Skill mix exercises have attempted to quantify nursing in terms of cost, quality and eventual patient outcomes. Trained nurses are vociferous when the subject of skill mix arises, but it is important to remember that health care assistants are much cheaper to employ than trained staff. Johnston (1989) suggests that managers will find it impossible to let trained staff do jobs that a health care assistant could do for a fraction of the cost.

However, as the report by the Royal College of Nursing has shown, untrained staff actually have more days off through sickness and/or absence per year. Therefore, it may not be cheaper to employ them than trained staff. It could prove to be more economically viable to employ more newly qualified staff nurses, particularly considering the high cost of training to become a registered general nurses.

In addition, National Health Service Trusts are now able to set their own pay scales and conditions of employment. This has led to local pay and conditions being imposed on new health care assistants throughout the country; although auxiliaries who have retrained remained on their old contracts. Clinical grading may start to be phased out in many areas as different rates of pay are awarded by Trusts. Local determination of pay could mean that health care assistants will be paid a basic wage for a certain number of hours irrespective of the shifts that they work. In practice, then, health care assistants who do not receive unsocial hours enhanced pay are cheaper to employ than existing auxiliaries who are entitled to such payments. This will disadvantage those health care assistants on new contracts, particularly those with family commitments.

Meanwhile, if the health care assistant is employed in part of the country where there is no shortage of people to fill the job vacancies, then the pay may realistically be lower than in areas where it is difficult to fill posts. In parts of the North West, for instance, traditionally the labour force is fairly static; people do not tend to move around from job to job and therefore it is safe to assume that the amount of people available for the posts of HCAs will be large. Buchan (1990) supports this by suggesting that rates of pay may differ widely in various parts of the country as a result.

It could be argued that when people train to be proficient at NVQ level two, they should be on similar salaries to other level two employees in other professions, as their qualification should be of an equivalent standard. For example, a secretary may train to level two of her occupational National Vocational Qualifications, but could be paid a very different salary to a level two health care assistant.

Another factor, when considering the health care assistant grade, is that when they reach level three of the training scheme their responsibilities will include more complex procedures and tasks, for instance dressings and recording of temperature pulse and blood pressure. This will raise the question of higher pay and new job descriptions, complicating not only the ward structure, but also the pay scales.

6. Level three – a new enrolled nurse?

Level three is considered as an entry gate into registered nurse training but it could also be argued that it will be the re-invention of the enrolled nurse role, one which the United Kingdom Central Council have sought to change by converting them to registered practitioners. Bolger (1990) suggests that health care assistants could be given a clerical and supportive role. He proposes that they should help to prepare the environment for the nurse to complete, for example, a dressing or preparing the bathroom or beds for the patients. He further points out that it is the supervising registered nurse who should decide what that health care assistant is able to do. However, it should be remembered that as registered nurses we will be held accountable for the mistakes made by the health care assistant when being supervised. Certainly not every health care assistant will be eligible to carry on to level three. The reasons for this would vary because some may find it educationally too demanding or time consuming while others will be satisfied with achieving a level two qualification.

The criteria for selection of staff for training at level three will have to be considered carefully if it is to be looked at as an educationally sound requirement for entry into Project 2000 training. It will also be costly in terms of finance and resources and for this reason staff will have to be selected carefully for this third level.

How do registered nurses view their role?

The introduction of the health care assistant should encourage all nurses to look at what they really perceive nursing to be. Is it holistic care given by highly trained, competent nurses working in an environment receptive to innovations in practice and research based knowledge? Do we want registered practitioners to be knowledgeable doers as discussed in the UKCC's Project 2000 document? Or do we want trained nurses to be merely supervisors and care planners shuffling pieces of paper and checking that the documentation is in order? No one would underestimate the importance of clear, concise, well completed documentation, but it is of little use if the patient is left in pain, has worries which they want to discuss or needs help to get to the toilet and does not want to trouble the staff nurse because they have so much paperwork to do.

Do we wish to discharge that 'caring' element of our work to untrained staff? That is not to suggest that the health care assistants are not capable of being caring and competent in their contact with the patients. Trained nurses do not have the monopoly on 'caring' but communication and contact with patients are an integral part of a registered nurse's role and we must be careful to retain it. The National Council for Vocational Qualifications, cited in a document by three Trade Unions (1992), states that at level two the 'minimum standard should ensure a competent performance under both normal and difficult working conditions with minimum guidance and induction and allow the individual to demonstate a degree of flexibility in adapting to new situations'. The idea that we should be expecting anyone other than qualified staff to work under minimum guidance is worrying. Most qualified staff would argue that to ensure patient safety and quality of care that we are all striving for, it will not be preferable to allow the health care assistants to work with only minimum supervision after such short training.

Giles (1993) describes delegates at a Royal College of Nursing conference in 1993 voicing worries over the reduction in junior doctors' hours by 1995. They were concerned that nurses would be pressurized into becoming 'mini-doctors'. Evidence of this is largely anecdotal, but there is a possibility that if we discharge parts of our role to health care assistants we will have to take on more of the medic's role.

In *The Guardian*, on May 11, 1993, Professor Eric Caines made what has become a very well known statement. He argued that 'amputation was crucial to the nation's health'. He went on to assert that if the Government were willing to 'confront controlling bodies of nursing and medicine the Health Service could be run with 200 000 less staff'.

He proposed that there was evidence to suggest that patients preferred to be looked after by support workers. This caused uproar in the nursing press, not least because he did not substantiate his claims with any research which had been carried out on the subject. It does appear to be the answer to a hard pressed manager's prayer – fewer trained staff and many more unqualified support workers.

Hancock (1993) replied to the suggestion that the National Health Service should have a greater ratio of untrained staff by citing the study carried out by Buchan and Ball (1991). This work demonstrated that patients recover more quickly and are discharged from hospital sooner when they are cared for by qualified staff. A study carried out by the University of York (1992) cited in Hancock (1993) replicates this research and reports that high standards of care were dependent on the employment of qualified nurses.

If Caine's suggestions were implemented what would happen to quality of care?

Consider the two following case studies:

1. Psychological care of a patient following mastectomy

A primary nurse has assessed that a patient returning from an operation would need careful monitoring of blood pressure, pulse and temperature to monitor potential postoperative complications. A health care assistant who, as part of his or her level three competencies, had been assessed as being able to record both blood pressure and take the patient's vital signs. It has altered little from the reading taken when the patient returned from theatre and so he or she records it and moves on to the next patient to record their observations. The health care assistant then continues to complete the same observations on another five patients who have returned from theatre. The primary nurse has planned that part of the patient's care and it is delivered by a health care assistant. That same patient who is having her blood pressure taken has just returned from having a mastectomy, she is frightened and upset, worried about her future and her family.

There is a danger that nursing care could become task orientated and the philosophy of primary nursing will disappear.

Have we all worked so hard to implement change and improve things for patients to allow this to happen now? A trained nurse, having assessed his or her patient, would be aware of this woman's needs and fears. While recording the patient's vital signs the nurse would be would be taking into consideration the woman's mental state, her responses to questions, her appearance and her manner, to name but a few. Skilled listening skills would be used together with counselling skills developed over a long period of time during post-registration practice. This holistic approach to care is deeply rooted in the philosophy of primary nursing and much more in keeping with the type of care registered nurses want to give their patients.

2. Physical postoperative care

In the second scenario consider the example of a health care assistant employed as part of theatre staff. His or her job is to escort patients back from the recovery area to the wards following surgery. Having been introduced to his named nurse and associate nurses on the ward, the patient is taken to theatre by a nurse with whom he is familiar. Following surgery he is drowsy and a little disorientated. He does not know the health care assistant who is to take him back to the ward. In the lift on the journey back to the ward the patient starts to bleed and his blood pressure plumments.

In the initial period after the operation the patient will have been cared for in a very safe environment in the recovery area. When he leaves that area to go back to the ward the patient would feel less apprehensive and vunerable if he were to be accompanied by a nurse with whom he was familiar. The other implication of this role for health care assistants is that it appears to make light of possible complications which can arise following an anaesthetic. One minute the patient is in the recovery area, surrounded by highly trained staff with anaesthetists at hand, and the next minute the patient is in the corridor or lift with a porter and a health care assistant. If the patient has respiratory problems or starts to bleed it is a difficult situation for a qualified nurse. It does not appear to be an appropriate role for health care assistants, but one which is being considered in some areas of the country.

It can be seen from these two scenarios that there is still a great deal of work to be done on appropriate roles for health care assistants. As stated earlier, nurses must be clear in their own minds about what they perceive nursing to be. The profession must ensure that the health care assistant role does not encroach on our own. The profession must also consider ways of expanding the registered practitioner's role to utilize best the skills and knowledge that are developing in nursing.

The issues raised in the preceeding scenarios are important to those who see nursing as something which should be nurse led and not politically driven.

In theory, the introduction of the health care assistant is of positive benefit to patient care. There are many advantages and it is vital not to lose sight of them in the midst of worries about accountability and skill mix. Registered nurses are accountable for their practice, and have to answer for their actions. Pyne (1992) believes that accountability demands 'a new level of determination to maintain and improve knowledge and competence in the interests of patients'.

While health care assistants are being supervised by a registered nurse they are accountable for the care that they give. However, it is important to remember the health care assistants have a responsibility to their employers to carry out work of a standard to which they have been trained. The introduction of the health care assistant allows the qualified staff the freedom to be creative in the care that they give to the patients.

It should not be forgotten that qualified staff were accountable for students before health care assistants. Care to some extent has always been given by unqualified staff both of auxiliary grade and students. With the introduction of the health care assistant, qualified staff will soon become familiar with this new grade of staff and will be able to assess their strengths and weaknesses.

Where next? Where will the future lead us?

Health care assistants have a very important part to play in the nursing team. They are valued for their skills and their expertise in the same way as every other member of staff. Many areas in the North West have more health care assistants than the number of auxiliaries that were employed in the past. This is due to the absence of students as a result of Project 2000 training. Previously, students were allocated to the wards and worked as part of the staffing numbers. With Project 2000 training they are not intended to work in this way and so there has been a shortfall in the number of staff on the wards.

Although it is important that registered nurses do not become merely care planners, the introduction of health care assistants has allowed the primary and associate nurses time to be able to practise their skills to care for the patients. The health care assistant gives care based on competency. The following examples are taken from the City and Guilds (1992) standards for level two which give the competencies on which the training is based.

The type of criteria that the health care assistants have to complete are, for example:

- 'orientating the client to the care environment' (showing patient around the ward); and

- 'transporting a patient from one care setting to another' (for example, escorting a patient with no major problems to theatre, or to another ward).

Each area of care is included in a 'unit' and in each unit are elements which are further broken down into performance criteria. It means that the paperwork tends to be extensive and this can pose problems for trainees who have a problem with written skills.

Health care assistant training is now well established, although it is constantly changing. Many of the existing auxiliaries have reached level two and there are new employees in training at the present. However, it is this second group who often find the units of competence difficult to comprehend. The language used in the units is complex and they find it difficult to relate to what they are practising in the clinical area.

Consider the following performance criterion:

assist the client to view his contact with the health care team as a positive developmental experience.

What is surprising with that example is the language used to describe the tasks that the health care assistant has to do. Furthermore, it could also be argued that if a patient comes into hospital for treatment they are not necessarily looking for a positive developmental experience – rather, they want their health problem diagnosed and treated. This example is used merely to highlight the importance of the training being relevant to what we need the support workers to be able to do – that is to give care under the direct supervision of the qualified nurse.

The time taken to complete the paperwork for the health care assistant is immense; they have an enormous amount of log sheets to fill in to record their practice and competence. The training is not intended to have an academic base and yet the written skills that are needed are considerable. It would be a great shame if potential entrants were deterred from the training because of the amount of paperwork to complete. Assessors have to read all the log sheets, having observed the health care assistant doing whatever is being assessed, and this takes a great deal of time in addition to the other work qualified staff have to do.

The course needs to be evaluated by people who are taking part in it, the health care assistants, the assessors and the training managers, to ensure that it meets the training needs of those for whom it is designed. This would help to ensure that it does not become both unwieldy and unworkable in terms of time taken to complete.

Recommendations

Nurses must ensure that they take an active part in shaping of the role of the health care assistant to meet the needs of the patients, the qualified staff and indeed the health care assistants themselves.

Patient focused hospitals have recently been discussed with a great deal of interest. Morgan (1993) describes the concept of patient focused hospitals as being introduced in 1988. The idea of having multiskilled personnel who can look after needs of the patient, thereby reducing the number of staff dealing with that patient, seems to be an ideal situation. Trained staff would be able to give intravenous drugs, take electrocardiographs and give basic physiotherapy so that the patient does not receive care fragmented by contact with several different professionals. Generic health care assistants who are able to perform a wide variety of tasks would also be included in this multiskilling and would work under the guidance of the trained nurse.

It would be very easy for managers to decide to employ fewer qualified staff and more health care assistants in order to balance the budget, but as has already been shown this could be false economy. It would result in qualified staff being nothing more than supervisors with the health care assistants giving daily care.

Quality would inevitably suffer, with patients taking longer to recover and patient satisfaction would decrease. Draper (1990) supports this view, saying that if nurses become merely managers of care, quality will decrease.

The advances nursing has made in the past years, through holistic care and primary nursing could be lost by fragmentation of care, task allocation and the confusion of so many different grades of staff in the service.

Caines (1991) suggests that the 'hands-on care of patients is below nurses level of competence' and that tasks such as feeding patients should not be the domain of qualified staff. Draper (1990) disagrees, believing that nursing expertise is needed for daily parts of care such as feeding and bathing patients and nurses should not allow those parts of care to be taken away. He also points out that if we delegate 'nursing' to the health care assistant we will be given more and more medical jobs to do.

Benner, cited in Northcott and Bayntun-Lees (1993), describes care as a 'dynamic theraputic function'. Nurses have worked hard to raise professional awareness and dispel sterotypical views of nursing. There is a risk that nurses might return to being doctors' handmaidens doing the jobs that doctors believe they should do on a task allocation basis – the intravenous antibiotics and taking blood samples.

Many nurses are already doing these things as part of total care of their patients and it is preferable that these should be done by qualified nurses. However, they should not be done merely as a task in isolation, as this will result in fragmentation of care. The profession should continue to discover ways to expand the role of the registered practitioner to utilize the varied skills and knowledge developing in nursing.

The rise in 'professionalism' for nurses has prompted more thought about what nursing is and how it should develop in the future. The introduction of the health care assistant grade has many good points and will be of great advantage. However, nurses must be aware of their own special skills so that they do not give up large parts of their role to health care assistants. Bagust et al., cited in Hancock (1993), assert that achievement of high standards of nursing care is dependent on the utilization of qualified nurses. Registered practitioners want to be able to deliver the highest standards of care to patients. Holistic care includes those tasks that are considered the most basic and these should remain within the role of the registered nurse.

A great deal of work has been done to improve student training to ensure that their educational needs are better met. They are taught about holistic care, nursing models and other innovations in practice. It would be sad if they were unable to share the excellence that they learned with patients because they have to delegate all the basic care to the health care assistants in the future.

References

Abel-Smith B (1960) *A History of the Nursing Profession*. London: Heinemann.

Bagust A, Slack R, Oakley J (1992) *Ward Nursing, Quality and Grade Mix*. York: York Health Economics Consortium, University of York, cited in Hancock C (1993) Fighting back. *Nursing Times*; May 26, **89** [21]: 18.

Barrett A (1994) Bendable or expendable? *Nursing Standard*; **8** [18]: 44.

Benner P (1984) *From Novice to Expert*. California: Addison Wesley, Menlo Park, cited in Northcott N, Bayntun-Lees D (1993) Who cares? *Nursing Times*; **89** [22]: 40–41.

Bingham S (1979) *Ministering Angels*. London: Osprey.

Bolger T (1990) Helpers are at hand. *Nursing Times*; **86** [33]: 22.

Buchan J (1990) Breaking away. *Nursing Times*; **86** [42]: 21.

Buchan J, Ball J (1991) *Caring Costs: Nursing Costs and Benefits*. London: Institute of Manpower Studies, cited in Hancock C (1993) Fighting back. *Nursing Times*. May 26; **89** [21]: 18.

Buckley E (1987) Student Nurses' Experiences of Nursing Dying Patients. A Qualitative Study. *Unpublished Thesis. University of Manchester*.

Caines E (1991) Vision or nightmare? *Nursing Standard*; **5** [12]: 18–20.

Caines E (1993) Amputation is crucial to the nation's health. *Guardian* May 11.

City and Guilds (1992) *Care NVQ Level Two*. Care Sector Consortium. City and Guilds of London. Department of Employment 1992.

Davies T (1989) Interview with Laurent C (1989) More questions than answers. *Nursing Times*; **85** [7]: 28–29.

Dingwall R, Rafferty AM, Webster C (1988) *An Introduction to the Social History of Nursing*. London: Routledge.

Draper P (1990) Change in nursing and the introduction of the support worker. *Nurse Education Today*; **10**: 360–365.

Fardell J (1989) Short cut or short change? *Nursing Times*; **85** [7]: 30–31.

Gibbs I, McCaughan D, Griffiths M (1991) Skill mix in nursing – a selective review of literature. *Journal of Advanced Nursing*; **16** [2]: 242–249.

Giles S (1993) Passing the buck. *Nursing Times*; **89** [28]: 42–43.

Hancock C (1993) Fighting back. *Nursing Times*; **89** [21]: 18.

Heenan A (1990) Playing patients. *Nursing Times*; **86** [46]: 46–48.

Hughes P (1992) The implications of NVQ's for nursing. *Nursing Standard*. January 27/ 7/Number 19: 29–30.

Johnston C (1989) Who is the support worker. *Nursing Times*; **85** [7]: 27–28.

Gann S (1992) *The Battle of the Nurses*. London: Scutari Press.

Morgan G (1993) The implications of patient focused care. *Nursing Standard*; **7** [52]: 37–39.

National Council for Vocational Qualifications (1991) *Criteria for NVQs*. NCVQ 1992. Cited in Trades Unions (1992) *You, NCVQ and Me!* COHSE, NUPE and NALGO. London: Centurion Press.

Pyne R (1992) Changing the code. *Nursing Times*; **88** [25]: 20–21.

Robinson J, Stilwell M (1990) The role of the support worker in the health care team. *Nursing Times*; **86** [37]: 61–63.

Rowden R (1992) More input required. *Nursing Times*; **88** [33]: 27–28.

Seccombe I and Buchan J (1993) *Absent Nurses. The Cost and Consequences*. London: RCN and Institute of Manpower Studies.

Trades Unions (1992) *You, NCVQ and Me!* COHSE, NUPE and NALGO. London: Centurion Press.

United Kingdom Central Council (1986) *Project 2000 – A New Preparation for Practice*. London: The United Kingdom Central Council.

University of York Centre for Health Economics (1992). *Skill Mix and the Effectiveness of Nursing Care*. University of York, cited in Hancock C (1993) Fighting back. *Nursing Times*; **89** [21]: 18

White R (1985) *The Effects of the NHS on the Nursing Profession 1948–1961*. Oxford: Oxford University Press for the King's Fund.

10 Building bridges: primary nursing in a mental health unit

Terry Keen and Pauline Weir

No two patients are exactly alike, therefore, no actual rules can be laid down, but the nurse will not greatly err who always remembers the humanity of her patients, and makes their comfort and wellbeing her first thought.

(Stewart and Cuff, 1918)

Introduction

The delivery of nursing care has changed considerably over the past 50 years. This has been an evolving dynamic process covering such themes as task and patient allocation, team and primary nursing and the more recent case management approach (Manthey, 1980; Waters, 1986; Zander, 1988; Merchant, 1991; Ersser and Tutton, 1991).

The essence of this chapter will be to focus upon primary nursing as a means of delivering high quality care in an acute mental health unit. It will begin with a review of the literature which looks at the evolution and highlights the developmental themes underpinning this practice. The author's workplace is explored and insight is given into why a primary nursing approach was adopted and developed. An examination of the beliefs, values, aims and objectives intrinsic to this change will be explained, as will the process which demonstrates how these were adapted to meet the needs of an acute psychiatric unit. Inherent to this process will be an investigation of the client/nurse partnership, accountability, responsibility and its relationship to professional autonomy. These themes will also be considered in relation to their application to practice within the milieu of psychiatric nursing.

Evolution of primary nursing

The belief in individualized patient care is not new within nursing. Care of a patient by a nurse throughout their illness was practised at the turn of the century by private nurses within the patient's own home. The private nurse cared for the individual and planned the nursing care required following consultations with both patient and family. Planning and delivery of care was on a 24-h basis and if the nurse was unable to deliver care another nurse, her associate, was called in. Private nurses were professionally responsible to the patient and accountable for their nursing actions (White, 1985).

With this in mind, it is important to establish how a primary nursing approach has evolved and make a clear distinction between other methods of delivering nursing care. To this end, five major types of patient assignment have evolved over the past decades.

Case method

The case method of nursing dates back to the beginning of the century, when nurses were hired by families to provide for a patient's special needs that the family were unable to meet (Schweiger, 1980). It was popular during the 1920s in conjunction with private duty nursing and emphasis was on carrying out medical instructions.

Functional or task method

In the 1950s with few registered nurses and only some practical nurses available, patient care was given by nurses' aides. In functional nursing, hierarchical structure predominates. Daily assignment of tasks to nurses is the basis of task nursing. The task requiring the least skill is allocated to the least skilled worker. The patient is exposed to approximately 12–14 different nurses each day (Marriner, 1980; Matthew and Serrell, 1984; Merchant, 1991). A medication nurse, treatment nurse and bed side nurse are all products of this system as functional nursing emphasizes efficiency, division of labour and rigid work patterns. Registered nurses keep busy with managerial and non-nursing duties while nurses' aides deliver the patient care. Although efficient, task nursing does not encourage patient and staff satisfaction (Marriner, 1980); however, it may operate satisfactorily during critical staff shortages (Schwieger, 1980). Finally, difficulty may arise when focusing upon the total needs of patient as accountability only rests with tasks which are designated.

Team nursing

Team nursing appears to be the method most widely used since the 1950s, but historically the system was first introduced after World War Two when there was an acute shortage of nurses for hospital work. Team nursing could be given by personnel who did not have the qualifications of a registered nurse but who would work under supervision. According to Marriner (1980), team nursing is a philosophy that supports group action as each team member is encouraged to offer suggestions and share ideas. When a team member sees their suggestion implemented there is both an increase in job satisfaction and motivation. The team leader plans, interprets, co-ordinates, supervises and evaluates the nursing care.

Nursing staff on each shift are divided into teams to provide care for a group of patients. Each team is led by a registered nurse who directs the work designated to the team by either:

- assigning tasks to the individual team members (Kratz, 1979); or
- assigning the individual team members to specific patients (Kramer, 1971; Marriner, 1980; Laforme, 1982; Matthews and Serrell, 1984, Babington, 1986; Waters, 1986).

Team leaders may assign team members to patients by matching patient needs with staff knowledge and skills and do work other members of the team are unable to perform. Team members report to the team leaders, who reports to the nurse-in-charge. Accountability rests with the care which may be given or omitted during the report (Kratz, 1979).

Nevertheless, both Parkin (1979) and Kratz (1979) believe this method to be fragmented and leaves patients feeling as if they are travelling upon an assembly line. Team leaders have expressed frustration at the lack of time available for providing care themselves, as the majority of time is spent supervising personnel. This frustration results in nurses becoming disenchanted and leaving the profession (Babington, (1986).

Patient allocation

Patient allocation ensures a nurse is assigned a group or case load of patients during their span of duty (Kratz, 1979). 'Nurses are responsible for carrying out the nursing care for that case load, with assistance for those elements of care outside their ability ... The principle of this system is to give total care to a group of patients for a designated period of time. While attempts to individualise care, continuity is sacrificed to the shift system' (RCN, 1992).

Assignment of nurses to patients may be on a daily, weekly or length of patient stay basis. As the nurse is accountable for a group of patients, fragmentation of care is reduced and the ability to plan and deliver care is more effective (Kratz, 1979).

Primary nursing

Primary nursing originated in America and was developed by Manthey (1980) within the University of Minnesota Hospitals in the early 1970s. It was cited in the English literature around the late 1970s by both Kratz (1979) and Lee (1979). Manthey describes primary nursing as 'the delivery of comprehensive, continuous, co-ordinated and individualized patient care through the primary nurse who has autonomy, accountability and authority to act as chief nurse for her patients' (Manthey, 1980).

Concepts which Manthey describes as underpinning primary nursing are not alien to nurses:

- Assessment by a specific nurse who provides day to day care until the patient's discharge or transfer.
- The primary nurse plans patient care for a 24-h period. Therefore, care is planned for associate nurses to give when they are not on duty.
- Patient involvement in both the identification and achievement of goals in relation to their condition and lifestyle is encouraged.

- Communication between nurses and other members of the health care team is promoted.
- Better discharge planning, patient teaching, family involvement and appropriate referrals are fostered.

In discussing primary nursing, Manthey and Kramer (1970) say it is a system for delivering nursing care and not a solution to all the problems associated with patient care. Pearson (1988) confirms this, stating it is not a panacea, but together with other factors can lead to a higher quality of care. 'At its best primary nursing is simply a way of organising the people on the staff and the work to be done in a common sense system based on professional organisational principles' (Manthey, 1988). These five principles can be summarized:

- Allocation and acceptance of responsibility for decision making to one nurse.
- Individual assignment of daily care by case method.
- Direct person to person communication.
- One nurse to be responsible for the quality of care administered to patients 24-h a day, 7 days a week.
- Head nurse acts as leader, clinician, educator, consultant and resource person.

(Manthey, 1980)

Nevertheless, Marram et al. (1979), Hegyvary (1982), Giovannetti (1986) and more recently Manley (1990) believe that primary nursing is both a philosophy of care and an organizational design. They describe it as not simply a way of assigning patients, but rather a view of nursing as a professional patient-centred practice. In essence, the beliefs, attitudes, values, approaches and perceptions of primary nursing create a philosophy for a sound care delivery system.

For reasons based on national or professional events, each system has developed at a critical time in nursing. However, the *Strategy for Nursing* issued by the Department of Health (1989), having promoted the development of primary nursing, acted as a pivotal role in its introduction within the author's workplace. Together with the wave of interest and enthusiasm surrounding primary nursing within the clinical area, the time had arrived which legitimized this approach in care. The next section will centre upon the experience of the author as a ward manager in a psychiatric clinical area based within Wirral Hospitals NHS Trust; and give insight into why primary nursing was developed.

Clinical area

A combination of both male and female patients with a wide variety of psychiatric and emotional difficulties were catered for within the 20-bedded unit. Patient care was delivered by nursing staff with a varying degree of expertise, and Table 10.1 represents the skill mix prior to and following commencement of the project.

The figures show the number of permanent staff allocated to the ward. First and second level describe registered and enrolled nurses, respectively, while HCA

Table 10.1   Staffing levels and skill mix

Prior to change	Following change
Grade G × 1 (1.0)	Grade G × 1 (1.0)
Grade F × 2 (1.86)	Grade F × 2 (2.0)
Grade E × 4 (3.86)	Grade E × 5 (5.2)
Grade D × 3 (2.5)	Grade D 1st level × 4
	Grade D 2nd level × 2
	(Total Grade D = 2.92)
Grade C 2nd level × 2 (1.5)	Grade C × 0
Grade A × 6 (5.2)	Grade A × 7 (6.13)
HCA × 0	HCA × 1 (0.8)
Students × varied in no. (approx. 4–5)	Students × 2
= 18 members of staff or 15.92 WTE	= 22 members of staff or 18.05 WTE

interprets the role of health care assistant. Alterations in skill mix were primarily introduced as a result of student status for nurse learners and the emergence of HCAs. Nevertheless, the review created an equivalent of two full time qualified staff which enabled primary nursing to be explored.

Two psychiatric consultants were attached to the ward, both having a separate ward round each week. Their junior medical staff conducted additional ward rounds together with weekly consultant case conferences involving the multi-disciplinary teams. Nurses, doctors, occupational therapists, physiotherapists, pharmacists, social workers, community psychiatric nurses, and where relevant the dietician, combined to form the multidisciplinary health care team.

Impetus for change

Before the author's arrival on the ward and prior to the introduction of primary nursing, care was delivered through a task orientated approach. Care planning commenced at the beginning of each shift and was implemented by several members of staff, who completed their tasks according to qualifications and experience. For example, the nursing auxiliary would assist with bed making, whilst the registered nurse administered drug therapy. Occupational and diversional therapy were minimal, trips and outings infrequent and both staff and patient education sparse.

In addition, the ward environment displayed numerous negative aspects:

- ward was in considerable need of redecoration;
- colour of the carpet was unidentifiable due to cigarette burns;
- paintwork stained with tobacco;
- an absence of pictures on the walls;
- no plants or other aesthetic decoration.

On reflection, the ward environment was in no way a welcoming sight for people already in a confused and depressed state of mind. Verbal and non-verbal communication shown by staff reiterated the negative aspects within the ward and was felt by everyone. This led to a task approach in care which was governed by the nurse in charge. In addition to the environmental problems enveloping the ward, care was medically dominated and service led. Little was done with patient involvement and therapeutic programmes were non-existent.

Two months had passed since the author's arrival, and during the fortnightly ward meetings staff expressed a desire to explore other approaches in ward organization and care delivery.

However, before formulating any plan of action or implementing any changes, staff discussed and analysed the existing levels of care, deciding what was good or bad about it. The task approach emerged as being very restrictive in care giving and professional development. Nurses were avoiding responsibility and remained unaccountable to patients. As Brown (1991) says with reference to the work of Menzies (1960), 'task orientation in clinical care arose partly as a social defence against the stresses and anxieties of the nature of the work'. This was true of the climate prior to change as the more senior the nurse, the less 'care' they gave. An individualized approach which continued throughout the patient's stay did not occur. Total responsibility for nursing care by a designated or named nurse as cited in the *Strategy for Nursing* (DOH, 1989) and reiterated in the *Vision for the Future* (DOH, 1993) was absent and required urgent attention.

Primary nursing in psychiatry

Literature relating primary nursing to psychiatry is not in abundance as in other fields of health care. Works by Green (1983), Ritter (1985), Bowers (1987), Blenkarn et al. (1988) and Armitage (1985, 1989, 1990) provided guidance and a point of reference for the author. As Green says, 'attempting to use the nursing process in psychiatry is worthless if the old attitudes persist ... what is important is the individualized, person-centred approach, planned and justifiable nursing; problem-related and goal-directed; nursing based on the clearly unique therapeutic function of the nurse'.

Patients suffering from a mental illness often require long periods of hospital stay. This is in comparison to patients with surgical or medical problems, whose length of stay may be a few days. In psychiatry, patients' confidence in the staff caring for them is a crucial factor in recovery. With primary nursing, continuity of care through a designated practitioner is encouraged and so patient anxiety is reduced. The primary nurse seeks to become the main carer, teacher, advocate, therapist, counsellor and resource for their client group (Nordal and Sato, 1980). Such differing nursing roles appear synonymous with the view by Peplau (1952). Although her views were written primarily for psychiatric nurses, much of what she says can be of use to those working in other fields. Peplau describes six nursing roles which the practitioner can use in the nurse/patient relationship:

- stranger
- resource person

- teacher
- leader
- surrogate
- counsellor

Thompson (1986) states that Peplau believed the relationship between the nurse and client could be conceptualized along a continuum from strangers to collaborators in problem-solving. The philosophy of Peplau's conceptual model for nursing and a primary nursing approach are both almost congruent. Both stress developmental growth and maturity of the patient and the nurse through the educative process. In psychiatry, Peplau's model can facilitate both the application and change of attitudes required within a primary nursing approach.

Finally, from a subjective basis, the literature offered a tangible resource and demonstrated a new approach in mental health care giving. Primary nursing appeared to create a more holistic and patient-centred environment and was therefore worthy of exploring.

Beliefs and values

Within 6 months the concept of primary nursing was discussed and debated. Staff had access to literature and time was available to visit other units which were pursuing the primary nursing path. It was at this time that the authors shared their expertise and pooled resources to educate the staff. One of the authors had previous experience of implementating primary nursing and within a current practice development role, was able to provide peer support and bestow a perspective from within general nursing. This educational phase culminated in a mutual ward agreement to develop primary nursing. They decided the aims of its introduction were four-fold:

- increase individualized care;
- provide continuation in care delivery;
- involvement of both patient and family/significant others in planning and implementation of care;
- increase both morale and job satisfaction for staff.

The first stage in implementing change involved creating a ward philosophy, which would underpin the beliefs and values in care giving:

- Care within the ward will be in accordance with the principles of primary nursing. Both patient and family/significant others are encouraged to participate and be involved in the caring process.
- Patient care will be delivered through a problem solving approach aimed at promoting self-esteem and independence in the individual.
- Following admission, patients will receive a fair and non-judgemental clinical assessment.
- Care will be planned with consideration given to the social environment of each

individual and the setting of both appropriate and achievable goals to meet patients' needs:

- In addition, care will be planned in conjunction with relevant social workers and voluntary agencies so that support networks, if present, are not broken down by their hospital stay. If these links are not already available, contact may be made on discharge to provide after care and hopefully prevent or reduce re-admission;
- Finally, based on the initial assessment, both care and treatment will be evaluated accurately on a continuous basis until discharge.

Aims and objectives

With reference to beliefs and values that provided the framework in which to practice, staff compiled several objectives for themselves to ensure the philosophy applied in reality. The staff objectives may be interpreted as follows:

- to work as a multidisciplinary team whereby care is planned involving appropriate agencies; and information and ideas are exchanged and shared;
- to support and encourage members of the ward team to reach their full potential and promote self-actualization;
- staff to be made aware of training opportunities and advised and counselled accordingly;
- to support and encourage learners on their placement and liaise with the school of nursing in all matters concerned with their welfare and education;
- to recognize and promote special skills and talents possessed by individual staff members.

The ward philosophy and staff objectives set the scene for the change to come. Six months had passed, with the educational phase in progress, when planning for the organizational change began.

Change process

Change requires the presence of a leader. In the present dynamic climate, the ward manager holds a key leadership position.

Historically, nurses have not been educated to take leadership positions (Irurita, 1988). However, Lewin et al. (1939) described three distinct leadership styles which are applicable for nursing today:

- Firstly, a directive or autocratic approach whereby the leader is willing to exert influence on others but is not influenced by them in any way.
- Secondly, the participative or democratic style may be used. This involves frequent contact with and influence by others.
- Thirdly, a laissez-faire type of attitude may be used which is neither autocratic

or democratic. Essentially, there is little contact with anyone and no influence exerted upon colleagues. In other words, a 'laid back approach' to leadership.

These leadership styles can easily be identified in nursing. A study by Baumgartel (1950) found that people working for a participative leader expressed a more pleasing attitude towards management than those working for either a directive or laissez-faire leader. With this in mind, a more recent study by Smith (1989) found that a ward sister/charge nurse's emotional style of management affected the quality of nursing. Management styles which encouraged a positive ward and staff environment motivated students to care for patients. This style of leadership is likened to the participative or democratic approach as described by Lewin and one which the author chose to adopt.

Communication

In applying a democratic approach to change, weekly ward meetings began with excellent attendance. The ward manager chaired the meetings and facilitated the change. Staff participation and involvement was encouraged to identify a strategy. Communication is a crucial factor in delivering quality and care planning became the initial target for change.

Manthey (1970) says that a well written care plan may not necessarily mean that the patient receives better care. However, it does mean someone has taken the time to utilize nursing knowledge, thereby increasing the chances the patient will have the planned care delivered. Nevertheless, Shulka (1981) discovered that better care may be largely due to differences in competency of individual nursing staff.

Despite these findings, a booklet was devised for patients and relatives which made it explicit that responsibility for care would be delivered through a primary nurse who would remain totally accountable. The primary nurse would be the main care giver and associate nurses would assist with care when they are not available.

Following assessment, care plans were developed by primary nurses, in conjunction with patients and relatives. It must be highlighted that patients may wish to remain passive recipients of care and no matter how enthusiastic and dynamic a nurse is, if patients do not wish to be involved in care then this must be respected.

Allocation of patients

Within the new system, the allocation of patients became the second priority. According to Black (1992), when attempting to allocate patients within primary nursing, several issues need to be considered in conjunction with their needs. 'These variables include the individual nurse's abilities, knowledge base and skill, off-duty patterns and annual leave, plus other commitments such as teaching, study leave or project work' (Black, 1992). She goes on to say, 'concentrating purely on the numbers of patients can be a "red herring" in the allocation of named nurses to named patients'.

This was true from the author's perspective. The staff decided to create four primary nursing teams, mainly dependent upon staff knowledge and expertise. Teams comprised of six nurses (day and night duty) caring for approximately five patients, allocated on a needs required basis. In other words, patients with specific problems were assigned to a primary nurse who had special interests and skills surrounding certain conditions. Two of the four primary nurses possessed a remit for anxiety/depression, whilst the others catered for alcohol/drug abuse and psychosis/rehabilitation.

Owing to this method of caseload allocation, it was acknowledged that some primary nurses would cater for more patients than others. Nevertheless, the staff chose the system as the preferred method of delivering patient care.

Role of primary nurse

Within the framework of primary nursing, nursing roles were the third aspect to be addressed. The role of the primary nurse has been discussed at length in many articles (Matthews and Serrell, 1984; Zanders, 1985; Kodiath et al., 1986; Mutchner, 1986; Black, 1992). They all agree on the following key remits within the role:

- to be fully responsible and accountable for assessment, planning, delivery and evaluation of patient care;
- operationally responsible for patient care 24 h a day, 7 days a week
- to include patient and family in formulating care plans;
- to use the nursing process in all aspects of care;
- to communicate with other health care workers on the patient's behalf;
- to plan the patient's discharge;
- to provide direct care to own patients when on duty;
- to participate on ward rounds and team meetings.

There is a plethora of literature commenting on whether primary nurses should be registered nurses. Mundinger (1973), Green (1983), Matthews and Serrell (1984), Zander (1985), Mutchner (1986) and Pearson (1988) all agree that a primary nurse must be a qualified nurse. Bowers (1987) and Wheeler (1989) stipulate only registered nurses should act as primary nurses. Meanwhile, both Wright (1987) and Salvage (1989) argue that nurses' experience and skills need to be considered.

With reference to the literature, the ward decided only first level nurses, (registered nurses and not enrolled nurses) would be primary nurses. However, as the majority of enrolled nurses were converting to registered status this did not present a problem. Enrolled nurses, nurse learners and auxiliary nurses acted as associate nurses, as did primary nurses for each other.

Generally, associate nurses take responsibility for patient care in the absence of the primary nurse. There role is four-fold:

- adheres to care plan written by primary nurse;
- alters care plan when necessary after validation with senior nursing staff;
- evaluates patient care;
- adds additional patient problems to care plan and plans necessary interventions following validation with senior staff.

Night staff are generally accorded the role of associate regardless of qualification, as the day shift has greater opportunity to liaise with the health care team (Wright, 1987; Manthey, 1980). From a subjective basis, the permanent night staff were involved in the development from the start and preferred to take on the role of associate.

Meanwhile, Wright says the role of nursing auxiliary changes to more of a helper, freeing the primary nurse from non-clinical tasks. They may assist all primary nurses according to patient dependency and ward activity.

The role of the nurse learner within primary nursing is also important. As Green (1983) states, 'if we are practising patient-centred nursing it seems logical to practise learner-centred education'. Everyone was aware of students' educational needs and objectives from the school of nursing. Learners were briefed on arrival regarding primary nursing and their role as associate. Each learner was assigned to a primary nurse who introduced them to the ward and identified any specific placement needs. The assigned primary nurse acts as an assessor carrying out the student's half-way interview and final report. Learners were encouraged to take an active part in patient observation, assessment, identification of problems, devising care plans and evaluating patient progress under the supervision of qualified staff.

Role of ward manager

Historically, the role of the senior nurse has adapted to meet the process of care. Johnson (1981) describes the ward sister/charge nurse controlling patient care by making all the decisions when applying the case method. They may function as a dictator during a task approach. Decisions are permitted by other members of the staff in team nursing, with the senior nurse retaining ultimate control. However, primary nursing allows the distribution of labour to facilitate individual patient assignment to one nurse with the ward sister/charge nurse acting as supervisor and co-ordinator.

According to Heslin (1987), the head nurse must create excellence in patient care and act as a buffer for staff, thus protecting them from unsupportive staff outside the unit and from inefficiency in support services. One must have courage to take risks and let staff learn and develop. Meanwhile, Sparrow (1986) describes three key remits in the senior ward nurse role within primary nursing:

- co-ordinating patient allocation and nursing staff;
- acting as a resource/information person;
- supporting staff professional and personal development.

Ward managers, known as ward sisters/charge nurses, are the senior nurse within a primary nursing structure and must, therefore, be a role model in clinical practice. Without doubt, the essence of change towards primary nursing lies in the ward manager and can be the key to its success or failure. Ward managers have traditionally been co-ordinators and planners of nursing care. Primary nursing decentralizes care and frees the senior nurse to take a leadership, consultancy, supervisory, resource and staff developer type of role.

Clarification of key areas within the author's role were discussed during ward meetings and focused upon the following remits:

- leading the planned change towards a primary nursing approach to care giving within the ward;
- remains responsible for patient care 24 h a day;
- co-ordinating patient care delivery;
- responsibility for auditing and evaluating patient outcomes;
- ensuring adequate staff levels and appropriate skill mix;
- establishing and maintaining effective levels of communication;
- ensuring staff gain regular access to continuing education and information;
- reviewing and evaluating the effectiveness of primary nursing.

In addition, the author adopted a ward co-ordinating aspect to the role as described by Black (1992). This involved having an overview of nursing activity; attending ward rounds in a primary nurse's absence; relaying information between nurses and answering queries when the relevant nurse is unavailable.

To avoid confusion, Black (1992) highlights the importance of role clarification when introducing changes in care giving. Differing boundaries of staff responsibility need to be emphasized and agreed by everyone to facilitate the success of change.

Primary nursing in practice

At present the authors have focused upon issues which encompass educational themes. The next section addresses practical situations which the staff encountered in the implementing stage.

Weekly ward meetings continued throughout the first 9 months enabling everyone to understand, internalize and adopt the changes. A major change during this period was the alteration in working times. Flexible working patterns were introduced and encouraged to ensure maximum patient cover was available when needed. A shift from the customary 12-h day to 7½ h reduced the likelihood of fatigue and sickness. Amendments to staffing levels and skill mix for day and night duty were agreed with both senior management and the finance department in preparation for introducing a primary nursing approach.

As a means of financing educational courses and study days, a training fund was established in conjunction with various drug companies. Normally, on the occasions they visited the ward, refreshments were provided for the staff; instead the money spent on food would be donated to the training fund. In addition, books, tapes, videos and magazines were brought for patients and staff from this resource.

Ward rounds

Consultant ward rounds were no longer conducted with the senior nurse who was on duty. Instead, the patient's primary nurse or associate nurse escorted the medical team and reported on their progress. As Green (1983) says, 'all team members (relatives, doctors, psychologists and remedial professions) benefit from the drastic shortening in the chain of communication'. He goes on to say 'they all talk directly to the primary nurse, who is the person closest to the patient and the one who can take nursing decisions'. Medical staff prefer to transmit information only once and appreciate liaising with the person who has a major role in caring giving. In addition, relatives can communicate through a single channel by speaking to the nurse who has complete responsibility for patient care.

Multidisciplinary case conferences directly involve the key carers. The role of the primary nurse ensures they do not waste time asking one person all the questions. Primary nurses are available for reporting about their patients; therefore no one nurse is completely occupied within a ward round or case conference for several hours. However, no situation is ideal and there are occasions when the primary nurse is not on duty and the associate nurse takes their place.

Before introducing change, drug administration was by the nurse-in-charge during a span of duty. Nevertheless, attempts to hand over to individual primary nurses have not been successful. This remains an area of practice which depends on staffing levels, sickness and ward activity. Owing to computerization of medication within the unit, the administration of drug therapy by primary nurses will be developed later than anticipated.

Accountability and responsibility

The essence of accountability in primary nursing is examined in detail by Ciske (1979) and Zander (1985). Ciske describes accountability as the state of being answerable; held to account for one's actions. A primary nurse is accountable to their patients first – and to be fully accountable, Ciske says, one must be a registered nurse.

When applying accountability within primary nursing, Black (1992) states it is useful to ask, 'Who holds responsibility for the quality of an individual's care during his/her need for nursing?'. In practice, the primary nurse assesses, plans, administers and evaluates care for a specific patient caseload.

Batey and Lewis (1982), cited in Black (1992), state 'responsibility is a "charge" for which you are answerable'. If responsibility is accepted by an individual then they are accountable for those actions.

Twenty-four-hour accountability was discussed within the authors' workplace.

Primary nurses were accountable to their patients, but this did not mean being 'on-call'. Associate nurses implemented planned care to ensure continuity when they were not on duty. The associate nurses were then accountable for their own actions; however, primary nurses were made to account for the prescribed care. Manthey (1980) says individuals who have been allocated, and who have accepted responsibility, must be authorized to handle the functions for which they are being held responsible and to decide how to perform those functions.

Professional autonomy

Autonomy means self-governing, and as Batey and Lewis (1982) in Black (1992) state 'it is the freedom to make discretionary and binding decisions consistent with one's scope of practice and freedom to act on those decisions'.

Within the primary nursing framework it gives primary nurses the freedom to assess, plan, implement and evaluate care independently for their caseload. Associate nurses may need to change or adjust care depending on patient needs; however, the primary nurse is informed at the earliest opportunity.

One may argue primary nurses are not completely autonomous due to the constraints within the organization. Nevertheless, it can be exercised as far as professional knowledge and expertise allow.

Benefits within primary nursing

Many authors cite numerous advantages within primary nursing. The benefits are numerous and can be summarized as (Shulka and Turner, 1984; Geen, 1986; Sparrow, 1986; McMahon, 1989):

- reduction in fragmentation of care;
- more time to provide professional and personalized care;
- staff inconsistencies in care are reduced;
- discharge planning enhanced;
- greater continuity and co-ordination of care;
- closer nurse/patient relationship;
- increased patient and family satisfaction with care;

Marriner (1980) found that primary nursing decreased the number of people in the chain of command and reduced the amount of errors that can result from a relay of orders. In addition, Green (1983), Lee (1979) and Sparrow (1986) believe that patients have the opportunity to develop a therapeutic relationship with one nurse; primary nurses are accountable for their actions, therefore inter-personal, clinical and leadership skills are enhanced; there is eradication of the care planner not giving care; and finally an increase in both student and qualified nurse learning.

The authors found many positive aspects after 12 months using a patient questionnaire (*see* Table 10.2).

Table 10.2   Patient satisfaction questionnaire

To help us maintain good standards we would be grateful if you could fill in this questionnaire. On completion, please hand it to the nurse-in-charge. Many thanks in anticipation.

1. Were you involved in your care?:   YES   NO
Comments...
....

2. Were staff available to you?:
      Medical   YES   NO
      Nursing   YES   NO
      Other (specify)   YES   NO
Comments...
....

3. Were your relatives given the opportunity to discuss your care?:
                                                         YES   NO
Comments...
....

4. Did you receive satisfactory explanations concerning your treatment?:
                                                         YES   NO
Comments...
....

5. Do you have any criticisms of ward facilities?:
                                                         YES   NO
Comments...
....

6. Was your discharge planned with you and your relatives?:
                                                         YES   NO
Comments...
....

7. Were you informed how long you would be an inpatient?:
                                                         YES   NO
Comments...
....

8. Do you feel you were treated as an individual?:
                                                         YES   NO
Comments...
....

9. Were scheduled activities provided, e.g. occupational therapy?:
                                                         YES   NO
Comments...
....

10. Do you feel your 'own nurse' has a positive effect on your stay in hospital?:
                                                         YES   NO
Comments...
....

Many Thanks.

Staff felt a nurse/patient relationship existed and patient care was less fragmented. Individualized care was the norm and an increased feeling of security was experienced among patients. Patients stated they preferred the new approach because of their identifiable nurse. Every nurse questioned felt an increase in job satisfaction as well as team spirit. New roles were clearly defined and access to in-service education increased.

Levels of staff sickness decreased from 8.5% to 2.5% within a 6-month period and the rate of staff turnover was reduced, giving more stability in the ward.

Access to therapeutic interventions in the form of group therapy were developed. These psychotherapy groups encouraged interaction between patients enabling staff to gain insight into the individual needs. Group therapy allows people to support and share advice with those suffering from similar problems within informal surroundings.

Finally, when relatives asked to speak directly to the primary nurse, rather than the nurse-in-charge, we knew the system was working.

Within 12 months the ward environment was transformed. The ward had been repainted with colours chosen by both staff and patients: comfortable refurbished chairs; washing machine; tumble dryer; television; video; stereo and various indoor plants were provided by the 'League of Friends'. A tape recorder to play relaxation music was purchased from ward funds. A patient information board was arranged in a prominent position to display ward activity and other relevant information. All this was achieved through an increase in staff motivation to improve the surroundings by asking and seeking management support.

Barriers to primary nursing

Laforme (1982) highlights several problems that may be encountered with primary nursing: caring for long-term difficult and dependent patients; discouraged team involvement and imposed nurse responsibility, to mention a few. Sparrow (1986) emphasizes stress levels may become harmful, while Ciske (1986) believes we need to prevent 'burnout' and so avoid the case of 'supernurse syndrome'.

However, it is unrealistic to expect no negative aspects within the system. The authors found low staffing levels during holiday periods created difficulties when allocating patients. Nevertheless, Cavill and Johnson (1981) argue 'staff shortages are a problem regardless of the method of nursing used'. They continue by saying 'this cannot be used as an excuse any longer and if we are to develop as a profession, we must practise what we profess to do, which is to nurse, and that means changing the way we work to meet the changing needs of our society'.

In addition, due to primary nurses requiring first level status, several enrolled nurses did feel undervalued. This was recognized as a short term disadvantage as all were in the process of converting to registration.

Another problem related in the moving of staff to other wards to cover unforeseen activity or emergencies. This was difficult to avoid and again applies within any system of care giving. At times staff need to be aware that a team or task approach to care is the only option, for example cardiac arrest or poor staffing levels caused by flu epidemics. No one system can be ideal but we can strive to achieve excellence within the constraints.

Summary

The authors' quest to improve care for patients is continuous. One may argue the changes are not unique to primary nursing. However, the system provided a foundation or framework in which to empower and develop nurses. The organizational change has taken 2 years to install and is in no way complete. If nurses are to meet patient needs, the way in which care is delivered must continue to adapt. Finally, in the words of Johnson (1981) 'If at first you don't succeed ... believe us, it's all worth it!'.

References

Armitage P (1985) Primary care: an individual concern. *Nursing Times*; **81** [45]: 35–38.
Armitage P, Champney-Smith J, Owen K (1989) Primary nursing in psychiatric care. *Nursing Times*; **85** [26]: 58.
Armitage P, Champney-Smith J (1990) Primary nursing in long term psychiatric care. *Senior Nurse*; **10** [3]: 4–6.
Babington L (1986) RN's involvement and need for achievement in primary and team nursing settings. *Nursing Administration Quarterly*; **Fall**: 43–49.
Batey M, Lewis P (1982) Clarifying autonomy and accountability in nursing service. *Journal of Nursing Administration*; **Sept**: 13–18.
Baumgartel M (1950) Leadership, motivation and attitudes in research laboratories. *Journal of Social Issues*; **12**: 24–31.
Black F (1992) *Primary Nursing: An Introductory Guide*. London: King's Fund Centre.
Blenkarn H, D'Amico M, Virtue E (1988) Primary nursing and job satisfaction. *Nursing Management*; **19** [4]: 41–42.
Bowers L (1987) Who's in charge? *Nursing Times*; **83** [22]: 36–38.
Brown S (1991) Philosophy for change. *Nursing Times*; **87** [30]: 59–60.
Cavill CA, Johnson JM (1981) Step towards the process. *Nursing Times*; **77** [47]: 2091–2092.
Ciske KL (1979) Accountability – The essence of primary nursing. *American Journal of Nursing*; **May**: 891–894.
Ciske KL (1986) Introduction of a seminar and classification of accountability in primary nursing. *Nursing Dimensions*; **7** [4]: 1–12.
Department of Health (1989) *Strategy for Nursing*. A Report Of The Steering Committee. London: HMSO.
Department Of Health (1993) *Vision for the Future*. The Nursing, Midwifery & Health Visiting Contribution To Health And Health Care. DOH NHS Management Executive April 1993.
Ersser S, Tutton E (1991) *Primary Nursing in Perspective*. Harrow: Scutari Press.
Geen L (1986) Cancer nursing: A special friend. *Nursing Times*; **82** [36]: 32–33.

Giovennetti P (1986) Evaluation of primary nursing. *Annual Review Of Nursing Research*; **4**: 127–151.

Green B (1983) Primary nursing in psychiatry. *Nursing Times*; **79** [3]: 24–28.

Hegyvary ST (1982) *The Change To Primary Nursing*. London: CV Mosby.

Heslin K (1987) Nursing unit changes from team to total patient care. *Nursing Dimensions*; **64** [3]: 27–29.

Irurita V (1988) A study of nurse leadership. *Australian Journal Of Advanced Nursing*; **24** [1]: 43–51.

Johnson J (1981) Primary nursing. Making a professional committment. *Nursing Times*; **77** [49]: 2089–2092.

Kodiath M, Cummings SH, Clementis S (1986) Primary care works. *Nursing Success Today*; **3** [12]: 17–20.

Kramer M (1971) Team nursing – a means or an end. *Nursing Outlook*; **13** [11]: 648–652.

Kratz CR (1979) *The Nursing Process*. London: Baillière Tindall.

Laforme S (1982) Primary nursing – does good care cost more. *Canadian Nurse*. April; **78** [4]: 42–49.

Lee ME (1979) Towards better care: primary nursing occasional paper. *Nursing Times*; **75** [33]: 133–135.

Lewin K, Lippitt R, White RK (1939) Patterns of aggressive behaviour in experimentally created social climates. *Journal of Social Psychology*; **10**: 271–299.

Manley K (1990) Intensive care nursing. *Nursing Times*; **86** [19]: 67–69.

Manthey M (1980) *The Practice of Primary Nursing*. Oxford: Blackwell.

Manthey M (1988) Myths that threaten (what primary nursing really is). *Nursing Management*; **19** [6]: 54–56.

Manthey M, Kramer M (1970) A dialogue on primary nursing. *Nursing Forum* (4): 357–379.

Manthey M, Ciske K, Robertson P (1970) Primary nursing – a return to the concept of 'my nurse – my patient'. *Nursing Forum*; **9** [1]: 64–83.

Marram G, Barrett MW, Bevis EO (1979) *Primary Nursing: A Model For Individualised Care*, 2nd edn. St. Louis: CV Mosby.

Marriner A (1980) *Guide To Nursing Management*. St. Louis: CV Mosby.

Matthews M, Serrell M (1984) Modified primary nursing to match staff realities. *Australian Nurses' Journal*. June; **13** [11]: 42–44.

McMahon R (1989) One to one. *Nursing Times*; **85** [2]: 39–40.

Menzies IEP (1960) A case study in the functioning of social systems as a defence against anxiety. *Human Relations*; **13**: 95–121.

Merchant J (1991) Task allocation. *Nursing Practice*; **1** [1]: 7–15

Mundinger M (1973) Primary nurse – role evolution. *Nursing Outlook*; **16** [9]: 642–645.

Mutchner L (1986) How well are we practising primary nursing. *Journal of Nursing Administration*; **16** [9]: 8–13.

Nordal DE, Sato A (1980) Peplau's model applied to primary nursing in clinical practice. Chapter 6. In: Riehl J, Roy C (eds) (1980) *Conceptual Models For Nursing Practice*, 2nd edn. USA: Appleton-Lange.

Parkin MMW (1979) Primary nursing: an american experience. *Australian Nurses' Journal*; **9** [1]: 35–36.

Pearson A (1988) *Primary Nursing: Nursing In The Burford and Oxford Nursing Development Unit*. London: Baillière Tindall.

Peplau DHE (1952) *Interpersonal Relations In Nursing*. New York: GP Putnam.

RCN (1992) Differing Approaches To Nursing Care. *Nursing Standard*; **7** [8]: 38–39.

Ritter S (1985) Primary nursing in mental illness. *Nursing Mirror*; **160** [17]: 16–17.

Salvage J (1989) King's Fund nursing developments. Primary nursing. *Nursing Standard*; **3** [35]: 25–26.

Schweiger JL (1980) *The Nurse As A Manager*. London: Wiley Medical.

Shulka RK (1981) Structure vs people in primary nursing. *Nursing Research*; **30** [4]: 236–241.

Shulka RK, Turner WE (1984) Patient's perceptions of care under primary and team nursing. *Research in Nursing & Health*; **7**: 93–99.

Smith P (1989) Nurses' emotional labour: Management styles affect the quality of nursing care and learning conditions in the ward. *Nursing Times*; **85** [47]: 49–51.

Sparrow S (1986) Primary nursing: organising care. *Nursing Practice*; **1** [3]: 142–148.

Stewart G, Cuff HE (1918) *Practical Nursing*. Edinburgh: William Blackwood & Sons.

Thompson L (1986) Peplau's theory – application to short-term individual therapy. *Journal of Psychosocial Nursing*; **24** [8]: 26–31.

Waters K (1986) Team nursing. *Nursing Practice*; **1** [1]: 7–15.

Wheeler D (1989) A process of change. *Nursing Standard*; **3** [35]: 26–27.

White R (1985) *The Effects Of The NHS On The Nursing Profession 1948–1961*. London: King's Fund, Oxford University Press.

Wright S (1987) Patient-centred practice. *Nursing Times*; **83** [38]: 24–27.

Zander K (1985) Second generation primary nursing: A new agenda. *Journal of Nursing Administration*; **15** [3]: 18–24.

Zander K (1988) Nursing case management: Strategic management of cost and quality outcomes. *Journal Of Nursing Administration*; **18** [15]: 23–30.

11 Freedom to grieve: a nursing response

James Brash, Christine McKenna and
Kevin Kendrick

There are few absolute certainties in life – death is one of them. When a person has died, those who are left behind can experience an emotional quagmire which is often given the collective term 'grief'. The process of bereavement throws a person's life into turmoil and crisis. A complex array of feelings can elicit all sorts of responses – rage, inappropriate laughter, silence, tears, thankfulness for a final release from disease, or, very occasionally, outbursts of violence towards the professional carers. All of this can play a central part in the close and frequent contact which nurses have with both dying persons and grieving loved ones.

This chapter will focus upon the relationship between nurses and bereaved persons. What will emerge is an exploration of literature relating to the grief process and how this can be translated into a pragmatic basis for giving support. This will be coupled with examples from the authors' clinical experience and detail a valuable development which is helping both practitioners and bereaved clients to deal with the complexities and traumas of grief.

'Nowhere to hide'

Despite the professional immediacy which nurses have to grieving people, research indicates that practitioners are often inadequate in the care and responses which they give (Hill, 1988; Morris, 1988). Despite such indictments, the need for nurses to develop a cogent approach to dealing with bereaved persons remains paramount. Archer (1991) reflects these themes by stating 'There are many reasons why it is important for health professionals to understand the process of grief. Bereavement is a time of great vulnerability and stress for most people, and is usually accompanied by a deterioration in physical health and in psychological well-being, which may in turn lead to other problems, such as hospitalization, dependence on drugs or alcohol, or attempted suicide'. Thus, grief is both traumatic and complex; dealing with it creates a vast challenge for clients and practitioners alike.

In a piece of extremely powerful writing, May (1969) proclaims 'Death is obscene, unmentionable, pornographic . . . death is a nasty mistake. Death is not to be talked of in front of the children, nor talked about at all if we can help it'. Despite the rather dramatic language which May uses, many of its sentiments are mirrored in contemporary culture. Talk of death, in many circles, still carries the status of a taboo subject and this often makes the expression of grief difficult.

There is a plethora of both classical and contemporary writings which mirror a constant theme of inadequacy in the way that practitioners deal with grieving clients. In a seminal text, Menzies (1970) examines the problems faced by nurses when they meet highly stressful situations such as dealing with bereaved loved ones. What emerged from this is that caring for a person up to death and then for bereaved clients confronts nurses with a very strong image of their own mortality. Menzies' research showed that nurses employ a host of distancing mechanisms to avoid close contact with dying persons and call upon these again later to circumvent grieving relatives. Kubler-Ross (1969) examines the difficulties which the human psyche has in accepting death as an unavoidable part of life and states 'In simple terms, in our conscious mind we can only be killed, it is inconceivable to die of a natural cause or of old age. Therefore, we associate it with a bad act, a frightening happening, something that in itself calls for retribution'. Nurses and bereaved clients share a common theme, a mutual and primal fear of death; relatives may be overwhelmed and deeply burdened by the death of a loved one, but it still mirrors the frailty of their own existence and the inevitability, someday, of their individual demise.

Morris (1988) also argues that nurses avoid grieving relatives because it reflects their own mortality. However, this research also revealed that nurses use methods of avoidance because dealing with the pain and distress of relatives demands passivity. This contradicts the traditional nursing pragmatic of always needing to do 'something with your hands' – seeking nursing 'tasks' helps to put distance between the nurse and grieving relatives. To a large degree, this hiding behind a veil of tasks becomes most apparent in situations where care is delivered under the themes of the medical model.

The following case study is taken directly from the authors' clinical experience and highlights some of the difficult issues involved in caring for people immediately following the death of a loved one.

Jill, a 36-year-old mother of two, was admitted to the ward via the haemodialysis unit. She had multiple organ failure and was desperately ill. However, despite her condition, Jill was able to enjoy visits from her daughter, Viv and her mother, Mary.

As Jill's condition slowly deteriorated it was felt that a side ward would provide privacy and intimacy. Mary and Viv were gently encouraged to bring as many of Jill's belongings to the room as they wished. The room was festooned with posters and photographs from family holidays. A hospital side room can never become a person's home. However, we hoped that bringing familiar and treasured objects would add warmth and vibrancy to an otherwise clinical setting. Jill's 9-year-old daughter, Pauline, could not bear to see her mum so ill and never visited the ward; Jill was always clinging to a picture of Pauline and confided in staff that she really missed her.

One Wednesday evening, Jill's condition drastically deteriorated. On Thursday morning it became clear that Jill would probably die. Sitting listening to Mary, she shared with us that another of her daughters had died 10 years earlier and this still caused her tremendous pain. Jill and she had struggled through that time together – the thought of a future without Jill was just too much to take.

Jill died at 11.30 that morning with Mary and Viv at her side. There was an immense feeling of sorrow on the ward. Mary and Viv were taken into the ward office and offered the customary cup of tea – together with genuine, but awkward, sympathy. Staff believed that distracting the relatives in this way would give an opportunity to 'tidy' the room and make Jill look more comfortable. They were then handed the standard piece of paper on how to register a death. Viv and Mary went home – ward routine continued. We began to question our ability to cope with the intensity and trauma of caring for the acutely bereaved person, and with our own feelings of loss about Jill's death – we had done our best, hadn't we?

In discussions following Jill's death, a number of key issues were raised about feelings of inadequacy in caring for dying and bereaved people:

1   Some nurses had found it extremely difficult to care for a young woman who had so much to live for. This had led to some nurses avoiding Jill altogether. Further conversations revealed that some nurses identified similarities with Jill's life and their own – this was painful and put forward as another reason for avoiding her.
2   Nurses expressed a collective fear of being unable to cope with questions which Jill may have raised about her impending death; this was another reason why nurses felt uncomfortable with anything other than superficial conversations.
3   Another source of fear was communicating with Jill's family about her death; as one member of the team put it 'What do you say to a 15-year-old girl whose mother is about to die?'

Some members of the team felt there was an imperative need to improve knowledge and skills associated with bereavement. This led to a literature search relating to these themes. The main elements of this search have been collated into a educational package which was given to all team members. What follows is a synthesis between the main points of the literature search and the practicalities of caring for grieving people.

Enright (1987a) quotes the eloquent and insightful words of an American student nurse approaching her own death: 'If only we could be honest, both admit our fears, touch one another. If you really care, would you lose so much of your valuable professionalism if you had cried with me? Just person to person? Then, it might not be so hard to die, in a hospital, with friends close to me'. Although this young nurse is talking about herself, the ethos of the words could make a resonant appeal for similar qualities to be employed in the care which is given to grieving loved ones. There is no doubt that caring for a dying patient can sometimes leave us, as nurses, feeling a great sense of inadequacy and loss. If nurses did feel safe enough to admit their fears and cry with relatives, professionalism would be enhanced and the weight of grief shared. To achieve this much would break down so many barriers and perhaps, just maybe, the words of the dying student nurse could be paraphrased to reflect the feelings of a grieving loved one:

'Then, it might not be so hard to *cry*, in a hospital, with friends close to me'.

The dynamics of grief

As nurses, we most commonly encounter grief in the relatives or friends of a client who has just died. However, people who are admitted with illness may also be in the process of grieving. When this happens the person's vulnerability is extremely pronounced because of the dual effect of illness and bereavement. This can happen with clients at any time in the life cycle but is a particularly frequent occurrence in caring for elderly people. What can be so disturbing about grief in the elderly is the cultural misnomer that it is somehow easier to cope with than when one is younger. Terms such as 'he had a good innings', 'we can't live forever' or 'we have all got to go sometime' do nothing to ease the tremendous pain which grief brings with it. Just because ageing brings an ever increasing probability of death, it does not lessen the sense of mourning for those who are left behind. In his famous poem 'Do not go gentle into that good night', Dylan Thomas, quoted in Enright (1987b), pours scorn on the perspective that, with age, death is more acceptable or that life has less intrinsic value by saying:

Do not go gentle into that good night,
Old age should burn and rave at the close of day;
Rage, rage against the dying of the light.

When death strikes it can leave a trail of grief and sorrow. A huge amount of literature exists to explain the key themes in the grief process. A recurring theme in research is that perhaps a sense of disbelief and unreality are among the most frequently seen, initial responses to grief.

'It's just a bad dream'

People experiencing the first traumas of grief often express difficulty in accepting that a death has actually taken place. Grieving people use many different terms to describe a sense of unreality and disbelief: 'this is just a bad dream', 'I feel like I'm outside of myself looking down on this', 'none of it feels real' or 'any minute now he will just wake up' all reflect the ways in which the feeling of numbness is conveyed. Parkes (1986) argues that individuals spend a lifetime developing a perception of the world which is based upon stability and permanency. The death of a loved one shatters such themes and creates a sense of turmoil and despair. Parkes refers to the Freudian notion of 'defence mechanisms' to explain the feelings of disbelief and numbness which often accompany the newly bereaved person. The reality of death can cast such a devastating blow, that shielding behind such mechanisms at least offers a tentative buffer from the full thrust of what has happened.

The anger of despair

The human condition has two primal reactions for dealing with threatening situations – fight or flight. We have already discussed the sense of numbness and unreality which some people experience; this is one way in which the psyche can seek 'flight' from the traumas of grief. However, some people react in terms of aggressive or even violent behaviour. This bears testimony to the power of the fight or flight principle in relation to self preservation.

As nurses, we are often the first people to whom the bereaved person has access to and may be the focus for a host of powerful emotions or actions. Commenting upon the potency of anger, Leick and Davidsen-Nielsen (1991) state 'Part of the anger which a grieving person expresses can therefore be understood as a "holding on to" anger. As long as, rightly or wrongly, someone is able in their mind to blame the doctors, the nurses, the ambulance men for not doing the right thing, then the dead person is, in a way, not quite gone. There is still a magic possibility that what has happened can be changed'.

The great paradox of anger is that it can create, for the bereaved, a cushion to soften the often unbearable impact of grief. However, when anger is directed against us, the carers, it can seem both unjust and unfair. Even when seen in the context of grief, it is never easy to accept the anger of relatives; it can leave us feeling assailed and vulnerable. However, dealing with anger is less traumatic than confronting rage. When relatives express fury as a part of grief it can have devastating consequences.

One of the most explosive experiences we have dealt with in practice concerned the father of a young woman who had only just died of an extremely pernicious, oat cell cancer of the lung. The man had been a member of an archaeological party working in central Africa. Members of the family had found it extremely difficult to alert the man to his daughter's condition. This resulted in the man arriving at the hospital a little less than an hour after his daughter's death.

A nurse accompanied the man into his daughter's room where the rest of the immediate family were gathered. As soon as the man saw his daughter he went into an inconsolable fit of rage; this culminated in a chair being thrown through the window and the man hitting his head repeatedly against the wall. A nurse was struck in the face trying to restrain the man and, as a result, was off work for a week. The man was taken out of the room by his son with the help of a male nurse.

A week after his daughter's funeral, the man returned to the ward with a massive bouquet of flowers for the nurse he had struck and two boxes of chocolates in thanks for the care his daughter had received. He was extremely remorseful about his actions and said 'I don't know why I couldn't control myself, something inside just snapped and I had to lash out – I'm really sorry'. Rage can be easily understood as part of an individual's immediate reaction to grief; it is less easy to accept when you are the focus of such a turbulent fury. Wright (1991) comments about such frightening occurrences by stating 'Rage is much more a physical expression and its release is usually damaging. In grief, rage adds to the torment and is a terrifying experience for the carer'.

The first savage cuts of grief can, as we have explored, cause a number of reactions in people; numbness, disbelief, anxiety, anger and rage are all part of the complex scenarios which can occur following the death of a loved one. However, although these reactions are what nurses may witness in the acute stage of grief, it does not tell us about the other elements involved in the grief process. If we are to understand and care for clients who may be beyond the initial phase of grief then research relating to other aspects of the process must be explored and applied.

A time to cry

Just as we are secretly aware from an early age that all things come to an end – then we become increasingly aware of the mortal nature of being human. This process of enlightenment may be gradual, which is why young children tend to conceptualize death in terms of a long 'sleep' and 'going to heaven', but there is an eventual dawning that we must all face death as an inevitable part of life. Reflecting this theme, (Kendrick, 1992) states 'whilst all of our lives have elements of loss, there is nothing which can prepare us for the ultimate of losses – the loss of self through death or the death of a life partner'.

Parkes (1975) has identified a number of major features which may be found in many reactions to the loss of a loved one. These are:

- A process of realization – denial – avoidance leading towards acceptance.
- Alarm reaction – anxiety, restlessness, fear.
- Urge to search and find the lost person.
- Anger and guilt.
- Feelings of internal loss of self or mutilation.
- Identification phenomena with the dead person – feeling close or near to them.

Parkes does not argue that all of these stages must be gone through before grief is complete, or that an individual will experience all of these sensations and feelings – it is simply a guide to the many facets of grief which people may experience.

Worden (1983) also sees grieving as having recognizable stages. However, rather than calling them stages, which he believes implies a passive response, he calls them 'tasks'. These he defines as follows:

- To accept the reality of loss. Denying the death of a loved one can lead to the illusion that death has not occurred. It is only when the grieving person accepts the death that the process of readjustment and acceptance can begin.
- To experience pain and grief. Wanting to avoid the pain of grief is perfectly natural. Bereaved individuals and those close to them may try and distance themselves from the pain in the hope that it may, in some way, be short-circuited. However, avoidance behaviour may lead to deep-seated problems in the future. Ultimately, there is nowhere to hide from the pain of grief, it simply has to be faced.
- To adjust to a new environment. The death of a loved one thrusts the bereaved person into a strange and unfamiliar world. Suddenly the house which has been

a home for many years can seem like a cold and empty cavern. This is because the person who helped to give it essence, warmth and meaning has died. Adjusting to a world without the dead person is a central 'task' for the bereaved.

* To withdraw emotional energy and invest in other relationships. This is the final task and is concerned with the bereaved person developing a social milieu which does not depend solely on the memories of a dead loved one. It is the final task of detachment in the search for healing.

The experience of grief is deeply personal and unique; it is impossible to present a number of stages and expect each bereaved person to fit the prescribed pattern. However, although research into the nature of grief does not provide a template for individual reactions, it can offer carers insight and clues about the tribulations involved. As nurses, we sometimes meet clients who are some way into the process of grieving. We recently cared for an elderly man, George, who had lost his wife 3 months earlier. He was admitted for investigations of weakness down his left side and progressive forgetfulness. During conversations with George, he would keep saying that 'Mary' had not been to see him and he was worried about her well being. When asked who 'Mary' was, George just smiled and said 'I'll introduce you when she gets here'.

Staff were puzzled by this constant referral to an elusive 'Mary' and we decided to tentatively ask George's daughter, Jill, if she would mind telling us who 'Mary' was. 'Oh, that's Mum, Dad has never really been able to face her being dead so we just go along with him now'. We gently spent time with Jill and tried to explain that George would have to accept that Mary was dead before he could begin to deal with grief. Jill was reluctant to accept what we were saying, feeling that it would be cruel to put her father through such a painful experience. We tried to reassure Jill by arguing that it was George's denial of Mary's death which needed to be dealt with as much as his physical problems; indeed, that there may even be a connection between the two.

In her own time and with the support of her husband and brother, Jill gently broached the subject of her mother's death. At first, George refused to listen and asked them all to leave. However, they persisted and, Jill told us later, George eventually hugged her closely and wept. The weeping slowly became a torrent of tears as George uttered 'I want her back, I can't bear this, please God no, please give her back'.

George was discharged 5 days later. Investigations revealed no physical reason for his forgetfulness or left-sided weakness. We cannot say there was a definite causal link between George's symptoms and the suppression of grief – but he has not returned to us with the same presenting problems.

Support and information

Caring for people like George emphasizes the need for nurses to understand the dynamics of grief and how it can present itself in a host of different guises and situations in practice. Reflecting upon the studies and research which has been carried out on grief and bereavement can offer nurses a rich base for creating innovative approaches to their own practice. In our particular case, the level of information available to bereaved people following the death of a loved one was totally inadequate. To try and address this situation, a leaflet was produced which offered a gentle resume of what grief may involve and a list of agencies which offered practical help (*see* Fig. 11.1).

A copy of the leaflet is made available to all bereaved people who have dealings with the ward. This is coupled with a personalized letter of condolence from a practitioner who has been directly involved with giving care and support. The letter always includes the ward telephone number and people are encouraged to ring should they feel the need. There is no magical panacea which can relieve the pain of grief. Indeed, as studies reveal (Heike, 1985; Speck, 1985) the processes involved in grieving are necessary and form a spring board from which life can develop focus and direction. Part of caring for immediately bereaved people is to create an environment where this process can be started and facilitated.

Facilitating grief

Hill (1988) cites the work of Worden (1983) as a means of facilitating the expression of grief. What emerges from this is a series of principles which can be readily applied to caring for people in the acute stages of grief:

1 Let the person talk, to help them realize the loss.
2 Allow the expression of strong feelings – anger, guilt, anxiety, sadness, helplessness.
3 Help the person to cope with living on their own.
4 Help the person to let go emotionally of the deceased.
5 Allow time for grief. Contact the person at critical times, e.g. 3 months, 12 months, etc.
6 Reassure them that their behaviour is normal.
7 Treat them as an individual.
8 Provide support over time, refer on to relevant support group.
9 Watch for maladaptive reactions such as the use of drugs or alcohol.
10 Refer for more specialized help if abnormal reactions begin to occur.

However, part of caring for grieving people must be to know our limitations and to put the time available to its most effective use. Reflecting the importance of knowing when to stop involvement with grieving loved ones, Morris (1988) states 'Ultimately, a great deal of undirected involvement benefits no one. For instance, the nurse may seem to hold out the promise of support she is in no position to give. Or she may simply become exhausted'. Penson (1990) gives a number of concrete and achievable responses which nurses may offer to people who have been cast into the immediate throws of grief:

Grieving – how may it feel?

Bereavement is something that most of us feel at some time in our lives. Bereavement can be a lonely and frightening experience. You may find it very hard to accept your loss. Also, you may find yourself feeling many different emotions which can be very confusing.

Grief is an individual process and we all react differently. We must grieve for those who have died so that we may go on living.

Here is some information that we hope you may find useful, there also follows the addresses of organizations which may be of some help to you.

Detachment

At first you may feel numb, almost like the loss is some else's, rather like looking in on someone else's situation. It is possible that you do not fully believe that your loved one has died.

Anger

Anger is an emotion common to grieving. You may feel anger toward your loved one for leaving you, at friends and relatives for being happy and continuing their normal lives, at God for taking your loved one away, anger at nurses and doctors for not doing enough and anger at yourself for the things you said or always meant to say and didn't.

Yearning

This is an emotion that seems to effect all bereaved people. Some describe this feeling as one similar to 'losing your mind'. For instance, you may think that you have seen your loved one in a crowd, you may think that you have seen them on a bus or even heard their voice, although you know that they are dead.

Health

You may feel tired but unable to sleep. You may feel hungry at times but unable to eat. You can find that you only have a short span of concentration and that you are easily distracted. Simple problems may be viewed out of all proportion. Sometimes you may be lethargic, experiencing aches and pains that you do not normally suffer. Whilst this may be a part of your grieving you must not be afraid to seek advise from your GP.

Loneliness

If you and your loved one had been living as a couple, your home will seem very empty and the feeling of isolation can be painfully strong. You may also find that friends and neighbours sometimes avoid you. This is because they don't know what to say to you and/or are finding it difficult to cope with their own feelings of loss. It may help if you make the first move, letting them know that you would appreciate their friendship and support.

Escape

Some well meaning friends may advise you to make changes, such as moving house, disposing of your loved one's belongings etc. Try to avoid doing this at such an early stage. There will come a time that is right for you when you feel able to make such important decisions.

Beginning to live again

With the passage of time things will become clearer and easier. You will find memories are perhaps less painful. You may find yourself wanting to pursue new or old interests. Sometimes you might feel this is disloyal to your loved one. Allow yourself to laugh, cry and be angry, you have lost someone and it hurts.

Try to remember, while the past will always be with you, there is a present and a future which is yours.

The following organizations are made up of people who want to help you and are happy to listen to you and offer their support to you. Some are also able to offer practical help:

Cruse,	The Widow's Association,	Age Concern,	Terence Higgins Trust
25 Hope Street,	Neville House,	5 Sir Thomas Street,	(AIDS patients and their families)
Liverpool,	Waterloo Street,	Liverpool L1.	52–54 Grays Inn Road,
L1 9BQ.	Birmingham.	0151 236 4440	London,
0151 708 5311	0121 634 8348		WC1X 8JU.
			0171 831 0330

The Society of Compassionate Friends (For bereaved parents),
6 Denmark Street,
Bristol,
B51 5DQ.
0117 9292778

Figure 11.1   Information leaflet

1 Make sure that family and friends are welcomed and listened to.
2 Be available to listen or just 'be with' the bereaved.
3 Answer questions honestly but with discernment and tact.
4 Offer refreshments – remember how dry your throat becomes when you're upset.

Building upon these themes, Morris (1988) offers a series of reflective insights which can be readily translated to the care which is given to the bereaved:

> We should not be ashamed to grieve and can often help others to do so. This is particularly important for those who try not to show emotion in public, which includes many men. All that may be needed is a hand on the bereaved person's arm, a few understanding words – 'you have every right to cry: she was worth crying for' – and you have given permission for the pent up emotion to be released. ... Knowing our limitations and, seeking support for ourselves when necessary, is to the patient's benefit. Sometimes, just sharing our grief with a dying person is the greatest gift we can give.

Free to grieve

This chapter has been an exploration of how one group of nurses has tried to respond to the needs of people whose lives have been shaken by the death of a loved one. We write about it in the hope that it may be of some use to colleagues elsewhere. The death of a client and the grief that results reminds us, as nurses, of the frail nature of the human condition; it also reminds of our own vulnerability. We have found that becoming familiar with studies relating to the process of grief has given a firm base for understanding the reactions and needs of those bereaved people we meet in practice.

Writing a personalized letter and providing a leaflet on what emotions a grieving person may meet has been welcomed by many of our clients. We do not have a formalized method of measuring the quality of this approach; however, its intrinsic worth and value may be seen by some of the replies which we have received:

> Thank you very much for your letter and concern, even though you are always very busy. To find time to write to us, for one individual person out of the many you take care of was very kind of you all. The vicar read your letter out in church and everybody said how lovely it was and that your letter alone was proof of what a nice person she was. We have had the letter photocopied so that every family member could keep one. Your letter has helped us in our grief.

> Following your letter, my father contacted Cruse and arranged some counselling sessions. I am glad to say he is now on the long road to recovery although he still misses Mum terribly.

> Knowing that you shared our sorrow has helped us greatly during this sad time. God bless you all.

> A special thanks to ward 6x at the Royal Liverpool University Hospital for the care given to our father and also the compassion that was shown to us.

These letters are not shown as accolades to nursing skill or the impact of the personalized letter and leaflet on the stages of grief. However, what we hope it does show is that we can all make an impression upon the direction and focus of a person's grief. Such a nursing response offers a key which can unlock and free a person to engage in the processes of bereavement. If we can facilitate grief we help the person take the first step towards healing.

References

Archer J (1991) The process of grief: a selective review. *Journal of Advances in Health and Nursing Care*; **1** (1): 9–37.

Enright J (ed.) (1987a) *The Oxford Book Of Death.* Oxford: Oxford University Press, p 77.

Enright J (ed.) (1987b) *The Oxford Book of Death.* Oxford: Oxford University Press, p 38.

Heicke E (1985) *A Question of Grief.* London: Hodder Christian Paperbacks.

Hill J (1988) Bereavement care. In: Wilson-Barnett J, Raiman J (eds) *Nursing Issues and Research in Terminal Care.* Chichester: John Wiley.

Kendrick K (1992) *Responses to Illness.* Disbury: Open College Press, p 62.

Kubler-Ross E (1969) *On Death and Dying.* London: Tavistock Publications, p 2.

Leick N, Davidsen-Nielson M (1991) *Healing Pain. Attachment, Loss and Grief Therapy.* London: Routledge, p 47.

May R (1969) *Love and Will.* New York: Dell, p 24.

Menzies N (1970) *Communication and Stress: a Nursing Perspective.* London: Macmillan.

Morris E (1988) Death and Loss: helping patients. *Nursing*; **3**[2]: 5–7.

Parkes CM (1975) *Bereavement: Studies of Grief in Adult Life.* Harmondsworth: Penguin.

Parkes CM (1986) *Bereavement: Studies of Grief in Adult Life,* 2nd edn. Harmondsworth: Penguin.

Penson J (1990) *Bereavement: A Guide for Nurses.* London: Lippincott.

Speck P (1985) Religious and cultural aspects of dying. *Bereavement Care*; **4**: 28–30.

Worden JW (1983) *Grief Counselling and Grief Therapy.* London: Tavistock. cited in: Hill J, *Bereavement Care.* In: Wilson-Barnett J, Raiman J (eds) *Nursing Issues and Research in Terminal Care.* Chichester: John Wiley.

Wright B (1991) *Sudden Death: Intervention Skills for the Caring Professions.* Edinburgh: Churchill Livingstone.

12 Birth rights: engendering excellence in midwifery care

Eileen Richardson

In an ever changing climate it is easy to become pessimistic and 'bogged down' in the mechanisms which have traditionally provided health care; providers of midwifery services are no exception.

Nevertheless, the last 50 years has witnessed dramatic changes in life expectancy. In 1960, according to Department of Health (1993), statistics within this country showed that 30 babies in every 1000 were stillborn or died during the first week. Meanwhile, the report states that the figure was less than 8 per 1000 births in 1992.

Owing to these improvements in life expectancy, midwifery care must adapt and change to meet client demand. Many of the needs women and their families have, are simple. They want care which is respectful, personalized and kind; familiar people caring for them; and to be able to make informed choices about treatment. They want a service whose priority ensures that care is focused on their needs and not on the profession (DOH, 1993).

Since the 1960s, antenatal care has been progressively medically dominated. The outcomes of pregnancy and childbirth depend to a large extent on social policies and organizations of health care in the country in which women live. In 1984, a report from the Maternity Services Advisory Committee, 'Maternity Care In Action' (1984) encouraged all births to take place within hospital settings. Meanwhile, more recently the House of Commons Select Committee, 'Maternity Services' (1992) and reiterated in 'Changing Childbirth' (DOH, 1993) argued that this can no longer be justified and women's wishes should be considered.

Drawing upon these themes, this chapter explores several innovative developments which supported and prescribed autonomous midwifery practice within Aintree Hospitals Trust in Liverpool. The underlying philosophy of the organization is one of investing in people. The trust believes empowering staff to develop practice has and continues to increase the likelihood of improving care for women, babies and their families.

Initially, insight is given into changes surrounding the structure and process in the provision of hospital antenatal care; highlighting the midwife as the main care giver.

Second, the setting up of a joint clinic for pregnant drug abusers is described; highlighting how antenatal care is given in parallel to drug dependency counselling.

Third, the provision and use of the first birthing pool within the region is examined, in addition to its benefits regarding pain relief. Finally, the emergence of the 'transitional care co-ordinator' role is addressed and its scope explored.

Antenatal care

Women often gain their first impression of local maternity services at the hospital clinic. The first visit is very important and provides the basis for future care. Large, impersonal, over-crowded clinics; excessive waiting times; dreary uncomfortable surroundings with inadequate or absent facilities to cater for children or women with disabilities are common. Such themes have a significant impact on attendance rates, especially if lives are already stressful. All this has serious implications for women considered to be at high risk in pregnancy. As these women utilize the service frequently, they are mostly affected by an inefficient and unfriendly service.

A qualitative survey of the author's antenatal clinic was commissioned by South Sefton Community Health Council in 1988. The study was carried out using a standardized questionnaire format by an independent company, Communique Organization Ltd. Patients and other visitors were encouraged to describe their experiences at the hospital with the minimum of questioning. If they did not volunteer information without prompting, they were encouraged to comment upon the following key areas:

- information received;
- attitude of personnel in department;
- atmosphere and decor;
- systems and waiting times;
- suggestions for improvements.

Results showed that the system of care was delivered in the following way:

- long waiting times – women were waiting for as long as 3 h to see a doctor for less than 5 min;
- care was dominated by medical staff and duplicated by midwives;
- women would arrive at the clinic and be asked to take a seat. Their name would be called, their urine tested and weighed; and return to the waiting room. Their name would be called again; escorted to cubicle to change into a gown before ushered in to see a doctor.

As a unit, we concluded it was time to shift the focus of service delivery from meeting the needs of the organization to meeting the needs of women, their babies and families. Improving the design and layout of the clinic waiting area would not solve these problems. However, it was seen as a integral part of meeting the holistic needs of pregnant women.

With this mind, two project teams were created. One team had a specific remit to focus upon establishing a welcoming and pleasant environment. Membership of the team included a works manager, design technician, doctor, midwife, accountant and manager. A second team had the clinical practice remit to develop care from a medical dominated to midwife-led, women-focused approach. The aims of both teams were threefold:

* reduce waiting times;
* provide creche facilities;
* deliver midwife-led maternity service and so release medical staff to care for 'at risk' women.

In essence, the project was envisaged to cost in the region of £75 000 of which £65 000 was secured from the Department of Health, whilst the hospital provided the remaining £10 000. The following section will describe the structural changes which created the new environment through which to deliver the new approach in antenatal care.

Antenatal clinic

Within the milieu of building alterations, antenatal care was transferred to an unused ward. This allowed the reception area to be completely gutted and transformed into a comfortable relaxing waiting area with its own creche. Individual consultation rooms were decorated and each assigned to a midwife whose name appeared on the door. All the consultation rooms had a call system fitted linked to the staff room. Midwives now seek medical intervention when women ask to see a doctor or if a woman's condition dictates. Doctors remain in an adjacent room and a light flashes, indicating the room number where assistance is required.

An independent consumer satisfaction survey carried out 6 months following renovations highlighted many positive assets within the unit:

* yellow facade of entrance door is welcoming and cheerful;
* open plan reception counter creates an air of informality;
* spacious and inviting reception area with harmonious and soothing pictures;
* informally arranged seating;
* well equipped playroom with nursery nurse supervision.

In addition, two waiting areas were developed to meet users' needs. An outer area was ideally placed within the entrance and provided access to the creche. The inner waiting area has seating arranged in groups outside the relevant consulting rooms which women visit. Waiting times, audited every 3 months, showed 94% of women were seen within 10 minutes of their appointment.

Amidst the milieu of structural change, a flexible appointment system operated taking into account women's individual needs. For example, appointments can be made with regard to public transport arrival time, women's working arrangements and meeting children from school.

Midwife-led antenatal care

Recent studies by De Costa et al. (1992) are cited in both Australia and the United Kingdom regarding the midwife's role. They state 'while midwives are qualified to provide antenatal, intrapartum and postnatal care for normal pregnant women, many do not exercise fully the degree of clinical responsibility for which they have been trained'.

Supporting this view, Robinson (1989) argues there are several advantages to care by midwives, with access to medical back-up for women. Care can be as safe as that provided by doctors and women prefer it. Care given by midwives has been associated with a reduction in the occurrence of a range of psychosocial outcomes in pregnancy. These include a decrease in the following (Slome et al., 1976):

• clinic waiting times of more than 15 minutes or more;
• poor ability to discuss anxieties in pregnancy;
• feeling poorly prepared for labour;
• lack of enjoyment;
• not feeling in control during labour.

Moreover, Liu et al. (1992) continue by saying there is a growing popularity among midwives to reassert themselves within their traditional role. They go on to state that not only women and midwives, but also obstetricians, are dissatisfied with the 'cattle-market' approach in antenatal clinics. It is interesting to note that Liu et al. describe the system as having been introduced in 1929 by the Ministry of Health to 'reduce maternal and perinatal mortality' (Ministry of Health, 1929).

Twelve months ago the author found one of the main concerns of clients and staff centred around medical staff. Clients were always 'waiting for doctor' or 'in the doctor's queue'. Many women were told that medical staff had been 'called to the ward' or 'still at lunch'. Apologies were accepted without criticism and there was no attempt to alter the delivery of service.

The climate has now completely changed with the whole system pivoting on the client/midwife relationship. The most important person is the woman, which is recognized both in practice as well as verbally.

The team which possessed the clinical practice remit consisted of doctors, midwives, social workers and managers. By securing a multidisciplinary approach, the chances of building firm collaborative changes are enhanced and ownership increases the likelihood of success.

Changes in care were simple, but had an effective impact within the unit:

• midwives no longer wore uniform but a combination of navy blue and white mufti;
• clients were encouraged to call midwives by their first names;
• clients were sent an appointment on receipt of the GP's referral letter;
• within 10 minutes of the appointment time, the client is called by 'her' midwife to the consultation room. The first appointment is scheduled for 30 minutes

(involving full history taking), while second and subsequent are 15 minutes. First visits to clinic include a medical examination, highlighting any problems and agreement to a tentative plan of care. Routine ultrasound scan and blood tests are arranged and discussed.

• clients see the same named midwife, conditions allowing, at every clinic visit and women can contact them by telephone should they have any problems or anxieties.

Comments from a registrar and midwives verify the success of the changes:

the patients seem to benefit from the continuity of care at midwife level and at the end of the day it is the patient who is important (registrar)

they have continuity of care as it's an all midwives clinic now . . . the patients aren't moving around, they come to one room. Care is based on patients' individual needs (midwife)

it's improved . . . there is job satisfaction (midwife).

In the study by De Costa et al. (1992) 'it appears that midwives' clinics are providing safe and effective antenatal care . . . 80% of low risk patients were managed by midwives with minimal supervision by the obstetrician'. The study concludes by emphasizing midwives gain greater job satisfaction within these clinics allowing obstetricians to spend additional time with 'high risk' women.

Finally, the 'Changing Childbirth' report (DOH, 1993) reminds us that 'Legally, midwives are able to practise independently. When a pregnancy is uncomplicated they are able to be responsible for providing and arranging all maternity care that is needed for a woman and her baby ... if abnormalities are suspected or occur, the midwife is obliged to refer to a doctor, and to continue to provide care working with the doctor'.

The success of the midwife-led clinic empowered and encouraged midwives throughout the unit to examine practice and explore other developments which would seek to improve care. This led to a second initiative surrounding antenatal care for pregnant drug abusers.

Care of the drug abusing mother

The lifestyle of women who are drug dependent differs from that of other women as their main objective is to secure enough money to support their habit. That is not to say they do not have a desire to be a 'good' mother should they become pregnant (Siney, 1994). Moreover, there is no evidence to support the assumption that these women are promiscuous as they are often living in a long-standing relationship, with the partner taking the responsibility for obtaining drugs.

However, pregnant drug abusers are often in poor physical health as drugs suppress appetite. Due to poor physical well-being, these women may have had amenorrhoea and difficulties with contraception. This, in turn, makes defining pregnancy much later and often leads to women only accessing maternity care when in labour. Even in these situations, women rarely identify they have a problem until perhaps 2 or 3 days postnatally when the baby shows signs of being ill.

Additionally, these women do not come forward for antenatal care largely due to the fear of having their babies taken from them. Furthermore, Siney (1994) describes 'the lack of confidentiality when admitted to hospital and the isolation and segregation that can occur when staff are judgemental' as another factor.

From the author's perspective, it became increasingly evident that the number of drug abusing women who were accessing the system only when in labour was rising. This led of the exploration and establishment of an antenatal clinic to meet the unique needs of these women. A midwife was assigned to manage the clinic who possessed both interest and motivation, over and above the positive and non-judgemental approach required within this specialist field of care.

Pregnant drug abusers clinic

During the period between November 1991 and December 1993, 83 women booked through the pregnant drug abusers clinic which was sited within the community. Prior to this, no figures with reference to this client group had been collated. Nevertheless, Siney (1994) states that preceding 1990, approximately 40 babies were born to drug dependent mothers within a Liverpool hospital out of a total of 6500 every year.

Following consultation with senior management, the specialist midwife liaised with the medical consultant who led the drug dependency team within the local community. A discussion focused upon the possibility of joining forces to provide a more comprehensive service to pregnant women in the area. It resulted in a collaborative approach to care giving with the midwife, consultant psychiatrist and drug team working together in close harmony.

The midwife visited the drug dependency unit weekly, taking the opportunity informally to talk to women as they collected drug prescriptions. Broad based issues were initially discussed with the women. As the midwife gained their trust and confidence more individual health relating questions were raised. Whilst health education advice was on an individual basis, topics were driven by the women or their partners. In addition, the midwife would inform women regarding Social Services support and how they could access the system.

A network of health professionals comprising doctors, specialist midwife, social workers and health visitors joined forces to work together providing a package of care aimed at assisting the woman to deal not only with labour, but with motherhood. One of the key advantages with this initiative has been the holistic approach. A main fear of the drug dependent woman is that her baby will be taken into care. The team gives women the opportunity to demonstrate a responsible attitude through attendance at antenatal clinics. This in turn, provides an environment for the woman to develop confidence in her mothering skills and prevent mother and child separation.

The package of care resulted in 95% of the pregnant women who were registered with the drug clinic accepting antenatal care. Of the 83 women who booked during the period November 1991–December 1993, 78 were seen by the midwife with the following outcome:

- normal deliveries   60
- caesarean section   5
- breech delivery   1
- premature placental abruption   1
- not pregnant   1
- miscarriage   2

The average weight of baby was 3 kg, with only three less than 2.5 kg and average Apgar score was 9 (8 pregnancies were still ongoing at the time of writing).

The specialist midwife caring for the pregnant drug abusers has the prime responsibility for seeing women and liaising with other health professionals. They have a responsibility to collect and maintain information and statistics which demonstrate the health outcomes of this group and evaluate whether the infant's health has improved. Furthermore, they act as a resource for other midwives, students, managers, health visitors.

Placing the mother at the centre of the provision of maternity care is consistent with other developments in health and social care. The crux of social care plans drawn up under the report '*Caring for People*' (DOH, 1989) is a needs-led approach. Unfortunately, combining this with limited resources may lead to reduction of choice and unmet needs. Nevertheless, by collaborative working, professionals at the 'coalface' can achieve much more by pooling information and energies rather than working in isolation duplicating each others efforts. It is hoped that expert intervention, at a time when women are more likely to be receptive to health education, will improve the health and social outcome for this family group.

Changes in antenatal provision having been discussed, the author continues by highlighting a dynamic innovation within the delivery unit. The section focuses upon the introduction of a birthing pool facility which provides water as a method of pain relief during birth.

Birthing pools

The first documented water birth is cited by Church (1989) as occurring in France in 1803. An exhausted pregnant woman is said to have climbed into a hot water tub where shortly afterwards she gave birth to her baby. More recently, Igor Tjarkovsky in Russia noted not only the advantages, but the beneficial effects of underwater birth for the health of the child (Jepson, 1989).

In Europe, the main proponent of water births was Michael Odent, a French obstetrician who oversaw waterbirths in Pithiviers Hospital, France between 1978 and 1985. In his studies, he claimed a reduced need for analgesia and a declined intervention rate for women who were allowed to labour submerged in water (Odent, 1983).

Over the years, many women have found comfort and relaxation in the early stages of labour immersed in warm baths. Showers and the use of running water have also been used to ease various discomforts (Lenstrup et al., 1987; Simkin, 1989; Balaskas and Gordon, 1990; Garland, 1993). Since these reports have been published, there is considerable interest regarding the use of water during labour as well as delivery. This is contrary to the lack of research regarding the positive and negative aspects of water births compared to other forms used during childbirth.

Meanwhile, according to Gordon (1991), despite few maternity units providing this facility, it is steadily rising as its popularity increases. This view is supported by Spiby (1993), who states that 'by now, at an estimate, approaching 1000 women will have delivered in water in the UK'.

In reference to this, Footner (1992) describes the use of water births within a Bristol Hospital 6 months prior to encouragement and support from the government (House of Commons, 1992). She comments 'the benefits to women using the pool as an alternative to pharmacological analgesia for labour appear to be immense. They feel in control and relaxed'. However, she states continual review, audit and research regarding this practice is paramount as a means of 'offering real choices in childbirth' (Footner, 1992). Interestingly, since the initial water births in Maidstone, Kent during 1988, all low-risk women are now being offered the opportunity (Garland, 1993).

Introduction of a birthing pool

From a subjective perspective, the first water birth took place in response to a woman's enquiry regarding the impending delivery of her second child. The woman had given birth to a son, 2 years previously following an uneventful pregnancy. Following much consideration and taking her previous obstetric history into account, it was decided that the unit would try to fulfil her wishes.

In order to meet the woman's needs, a pool was temporarily installed in one of the second stage labour rooms within the delivery suite. Several midwives were interested in this alternative approach in childbirth and provided the woman with professional knowledge and support.

Much preparation and enthusiasm was generated as both family and staff waited for the impending birth. However, the subsequent satisfaction gained by everyone following the birth made all the planning and effort worthwhile.

Following the delivery, several midwives pursued this innovation with rigour and determination. Their quest was to explore the possibility of continuing to offer this facility on a permanent basis as an alternative method of both pain relief and giving birth.

A short questionnaire was designed to identify the amount of interest there was likely to be surrounding the use of water in delivery (*see* Figs 12.1 and 12.2). This was distributed to both patients and staff, resulting in many women wishing to opt for water as a method of pain relief.

Aintree Hospitals NHS Trust

Obstetrics and Gynaecology Directorate

W A T E R   B I R T H   Q U E S T I O N N A I R E

If a waterbirth facility was available would you consider using it for:

		Yes	No
A	Pain relief	☐	☐
B	Birth	☐	☐
C	Both of the above	☐	☐
D	None of these	☐	☐

Figure 12. 1   Water birth questionnaire

As a result, in early 1991, a permanent birthing pool was installed within the delivery suite at a cost of £3000. Funding had been provided partly by a donation from The Women's Royal Voluntary Service, in addition to savings from within the directorate.

It was necessary to perform a structural survey of the labour ward building before installation, as a means of ensuring the fabric of the building was strong enough to withstand the extra weight of a large pool of water. The pool itself can be compared to an ordinary bath which is twice the average size.

Use of the birthing pool

The birthing pool became operational within the maternity unit in July 1991. Initially, women of low obstetric risk were permitted to use it. Only women with an uncomplicated past obstetric history and antenatal course reaching 37 weeks gestation, in addition to commencing spontaneous labour with a cephalic presentation, were allowed to enter the pool. The use of water as pain relief during the

---

Aintree Hospitals NHS Trust

Directorate of Obstetrics & Gynaecology

<u>Midwives' Questionnaire</u>

<u>Warm water bathing in labour/delivery</u>

Please answer all questions: If question not applicable to you please write N/A

1 Are you willing to care for a woman requesting to use the pool for:

   a. Labour   Yes ☐   No ☐

   b. For delivery   Yes ☐   No ☐

If you have answered no to either of the above, please give a brief explanation why ....

....

....

2 Have you been present at a water birth?

                             Yes ☐   No ☐

3 Have you looked after a woman labouring in the pool?

                             Yes ☐   No ☐

4 Have you conducted a delivery in water?

                             Yes ☐   No ☐

5 If you have been looking after a woman in labour and she left the pool in labour was it because (please tick appropriate box, you may tick more than one box)

   a her choice   ☐

   b a problem occurred   ☐

   c she wished another form of analgesia   ☐

   d you were unhappy to conduct the delivery in water ☐

Other reason, please state:

....

....

....

6 Management want to support you in caring for women using warm water bathing for labour and/or delivery and wish to discover your training needs. To help us to achieve this could you please state below what you feel those training needs are:

....

....

....

....

Thank you for your co-operation in completing this questionnaire.

Figure 12.2 Midwives' questionnaire

first stage of labour in women where the fetus is presenting by breech have been reported (Odent, 1983). However, to allow a breech delivery under water as discussed by Callanan (1986) is clearly dangerous and should not be practised.

When midwives gained the expertise and confidence to implement this practice, criteria widened to include women who had labour introduced with intravaginal prostaglandins, as far as their pregnancy had, until that point been uneventful. Women who did not meet this criteria, but still expressed a desire to use with facility were individually considered. Decisions were made collaboratively between the woman, midwife and obstetrician.

Criteria for good practice

Prior to entering the pool, a vaginal examination needs to be performed as means of assessing the progress of labour. Nevertheless, rupture of the membranes is not considered to be contrary to using the pool. Ideally, the cervix should be dilated to 5 cm (Milner, 1988; Jepson, 1989; Church, 1989). Moreover, women should not be allowed to use the pool if opiate analgesia has been administered within the previous 4 h. Should women require analgesia when in the water, nitrus oxide and oxygen (Entonox) is preferable.

As Garland (1993) states, there are numerous operational issues to implement safe practice, the first of these being fetal monitoring. During the first stage of labour, maternal and fetal observations are taken as for any normal labour. The use of a pinnard or water resistant doppler fetal stethoscope to listen to the fetal heart avoids disturbing the woman unnecessarily.

Water temperature is kept at what is preferable for the woman and she is encouraged to adopt the most comfortable position. However, water temperature is important to maintain body temperature of the baby and Garland (1993) suggests 'a temperature which is constant ... blood temp. 37–38°C for delivery and within 3°C either side of that during labour ... to enhance uterine contractions' is to be encouraged. Furthermore, it is thought that one of the main stimuli for the baby to breath is the change in ambient temperature, together with the change of air and an interruption of placental perfusion (Marlow, 1989). This being the case, the baby will not be stimulated to breath if the water temperature is maintained at 37–38°C during the second stage of labour.

It is important to ensure the woman does not become dehydrated whilst in the water. She should be encouraged to drink plenty and should receive adequate ventilation. The birthing pool can become both hot and humid, making working conditions for the attending midwife uncomfortable (Corbishley, 1989). With this in mind, staff need to adapt and dress appropriately.

Finally, lying supine with the head supported is not discouraged as the added buoyancy of the water prevents hypotension syndrome and reduces pressure on the contracting abdomen (Footner, 1992). Deep water within the birthing pool enables women to change their position with ease and adopt either a relaxed floating or squat position.

Second stage of labour

During delivery, directive pushing and traditional control of the head is not advocated, as this provides unnecessary stimulation to the baby. Footner (1992) says 'it is only when the baby is delivered that the midwife needs to reach into the water'. Once delivered, the baby is immediately brought to the surface and calculation of the Apgar score is commenced. The baby should never be held under water until the cord stops pulsating. A pulsating cord merely indicates that the baby's heart is beating and not that it is receiving adequate oxygen. If delivery of the shoulders becomes compromised, the woman should stand. If this does not facilitate the delivery of the shoulders, the plug should be removed and the woman positioned on all fours to bring about a positive outcome.

Third stage of labour

On completion of the second stage of labour, the woman is encouraged to leave the pool or the water should be emptied in order to avoid the theoretical risk of water embolus (Odent, 1983; Footner, 1992). Following the delivery of the baby, the uterus contracts, reducing the placental area by as much as 50% before the separation begins. The blood in the maternal sinus becomes congested and is forced back into the spongy layer of the uterus, thus further limiting the supply of adequately oxygenated blood to the baby. Such practice, if conducted underwater, will place the baby at risk of hypoxia (Page, 1988).

Withholding prophylactic oxytocin, absent cord traction and using maternal effort aided by gravity to expel the placenta, have demonstrated there is an increased blood loss, greater need for blood transfusion, longer third stage and greater need for oxytocin (Prendeville and Elbourne, 1989). These findings result in the third stage being more commonly conducted in the air using active management, for example early clamping of the cord, prophylactic oxytocin and controlled cord traction.

Finally, the incidence of perineal trauma is reduced in women who labour in water. It is thought that there is an increase of suppleness and softness of the vagina and perineum making tearing or the need for episiotomy a less common occurrence (Corbishley, 1989; Gordon, 1991).

Water as a means of pain relief and a medium for birth has become an integral part of the choice we are able to offer women. Recently, the Royal College of Obstetricians and Gynaecologists criticized the use of water by midwives, commenting on the lack of research to support introducing the facility (RCOG, 1993). However, such criticism can be levelled at many aspects of practice, for example episiotomy and elective caesarian for breech presentation. Nevertheless, Spiby (1993) claims two forms of evaluation can be used when examining effectiveness of water births. First, 'an audit will help with the trouble-shooting of problems in the early stage of providing a service, and with in-service training ...'. Second, she describes the use of both experimental (randomized controlled trials) and qualitative approaches to address patient/client outcomes.

Despite the poor but increasing levels of evaluation surrounding water births, it is important carefully to monitor practice and developments. Guidelines need to exist and be adhered to as with any other innovation.

The concluding section of the chapter focuses upon a fourth innovation within the author's midwifery unit. Insight into the multifaceted role of transitional care co-ordinator is given; highlighting the care and support for mothers whose babies are born either prematurely or with non-life threatening problems.

Transitional care

Transitional care was first researched and introduced within America in 1971, and brought to the United Kingdom in 1975 (Boxall and Whitby, 1989). A broad definition of transitional care from the author's perspective, means caring for the newborn infant adjacent to its mother in the postnatal ward. The problems surrounding separation of a baby from the mother are succinctly documented by Klaus and Kennell (1982), suggesting mother and infant 'bonding' is likely to be affected if this occurred immediately following birth.

A national survey carried out in maternity units during 1984–85 highlighted current practice with regard to low birth weight and low dependency special care babies (Dear and McLain, 1987). In addition, they considered the difference in hospitals practising transitional care in delegated areas as opposed to postnatal wards. Results highlighted that admission depended upon local policies; 17% admitted that all pre-term infants less than 37 weeks gestation were routinely admitted to a special care baby/neonatal intensive care unit.

The author's unit introduced transitional care in 1991, as an attempt to provide another option of care for a selected group of babies. Six cots were distributed, two on each of the postnatal wards, with the intention of providing transitional care to babies that would have traditionally been sent to the neonatal unit. Care of the infant was shared by the mother, ward midwife and a recently appointed experienced neonatal nurse – in other words, a transitional care co-ordinator.

Success of transitional care was dependent upon the post holder. It was crucial that the 'right' person is appointed with the 'right' personality and qualifications. Midwifery status is not compulsory, but a registered general nurse with ENB 405 – Neonatal Intensive Care Course experience is an essential prerequisite. Furthermore, Fig. 12.3 gives detailed insight into the objectives and specific remit of the post.

The postholder needs expertise to provide both support and education for highly skilled staff in their own environment; whilst having the ability to communicate effectively with mothers and families in a positive non-condescending way. Promoting effective communication links ensured that staff pooled their ideas and resources. This in turn maximized the potential of both staff and service as a whole.

South Sefton (Merseyside) Health Authority

Fazakerley Hospital

Job title:	Transitional Care Co-ordinator
Responsible to:	Head of Midwifery
Reports to:	Midwifery Unit Manager
Qualifications:	RM/RSCN ENB Course 405 or equivalent Relevant experience at B Grade Evidence of professional development

Objectives:

To abide by the legal requirements and (statutory rules) relating to Midwifery/Nursing Practice.

To promote and maintain standards of professional practices in order to enhance the quality of care for the patients.

To liaise between all health professionals on matters relating to Transitional Care.

To carry out the functions required to fulfil the goods and services provided by the Transitional Care Co-ordinator.

Functions:

1. Clinical

   1.1 To facilitate the setting and the monitoring of standards relating to Transitional Care within the Maternity Unit.

   1.2 To liaise with Neonatal Intensive Care Staff, Ward Management, Community Midwives, Health Visitors and other Health Professionals on all matters relating to Transitional Care.

   1.3 To liaise with the Ward Manager, Medical Staff and other disciplines on the management of the infant requiring Transitional Care.

   1.4 To visit the homes of babies who will have or have specific problems on discharge from NNICU or the Maternity Unit – by parental invitation and in co-operation with other Health Professionals.

   1.5 To promote the involvement of parents in the care of their infant who requires Transitional Care, and to give all necessary support during this period.

   1.6 To support all staff involved in the care of an infant requiring Transitional Care.

   1.7 To maintain a knowledge of the infants in NNICU and to communicate with their parents and to assist in any foreseeable problems relating to the baby's discharge.

2. General Management

   2.1 To assist in the development of policies and guidelines relevant to Transitional Care.

3. Teaching

   3.1 To initiate and participate in programmes of ward based teaching in matters of Transitional Care.

   3.2 To advise other Health Professionals on Transitional Care.

4. Research

   4.1 To promote a critical and analytical approach to the delivery of Transitional Care.

   4.2 To initiate and participate in research into Transitional Care.

   4.3 In conjunction with staff from NNICU, the Wards and the Community, to introduce and apply research findings to nursing practice where relevant.

   4.4 To facilitate the dissemination of local research findings on Transitional Care, throughout the Maternity Unit.

It is incumbent on the post holder continually to update his/her professional and managerial awareness.

Figure 12.3 Job specification for transitional care co-ordinator

It was essential that clinical staff worked closely with the nursing information office to formulate demand categories of care for the babies, as quality results can only be gained from quality information data supplied. Initially, mother and baby are categorized as one unit, with the possibility of changing as computer software becomes more flexible.

As stated earlier, the decision to admit an infant to a neonatal unit, separated from their mother, is frequently based upon the birth weight and gestation. This resulted in specific criteria for transitional care to be devised within the author's workplace and includes the following:

- babies who are well but need tube feeds;
- babies undergoing phototherapy;
- babies receiving special monitoring (for example blood glucose estimations);
- babies who need constant supervision as in the case of babies with drug abusing mothers;
- babies being treated with intravenous antibiotics.

Presently, five categories demonstrate the level of dependency and intervention required by the transitional care co-ordinator. The categories have been defined and redefined by staff within the unit. Data are collected at the end of each of three shifts, based on the professional judgement by the individual care provider. This approach has been accepted due to the lack of research within this field: however, it is open to criticism whether there is consistency in the judgement of patient needs. In the future, there may be justification for the separation of mother and baby as a means of demonstrating increased workload. From the author's perspective, the majority of babies fall into category four – babies with drug abusing mothers. This group requires greater educational, psychological and physical intervention from staff for the baby, mother and father.

As staff gain more confidence and expertise, more babies can be cared for within transitional care. This in turn, will create opportunity for neonatal units to concentrate on mothers of acutely ill babies.

Success of transitional care has been largely due to committed staff, especially the transitional care postholder, who adopted a flexible work pattern so as to meet the needs of the service.

Quality of service has improved, with mothers able to play an active part in caring for their babies as opposed to being separated from them by admission to a neonatal unit.

The transitional care co-ordinator, working both in a flexible and specialist field, acts as a valuable link within the multidisciplinary health care team. In addition to carrying a client workload, the opportunity to share expertise with other practitioners has reaped benefits on both a personal and professional basis. Integral to the post has been formulating standards of care for babies within the client group and participating in ongoing research reviewing babies of drug abusing mothers.

Steps in achieving excellence

The key to success of these and other innovations has been communication. Communication is effective when staff have the opportunity to introduce and develop their ideas.

Developing practice is central to a practitioner's role. As the United Kingdom Central Council for Nurses, Midwives and Visitors states in the *Code of Conduct* 'in the exercise of professional accountability' the midwife 'must act always in such a manner as to promote and safeguard the interests and well-being of patients and clients' (UKCC, 1992a). This theme is expounded within the *Scope of Professional Practice* stating 'particular developments may require midwives to acquire new skills because of the particular settings in which they practice' (UKCC, 1992b).

Managers need to capitalize on the commitment, experience and knowledge of colleagues. They must actively seek ideas from users of the service and service deliverers, listening to what they have to say rather than making assumptions (Rowntree, 1991).

Every organization must review and renew its public purpose from time to time. We should not ignore the clear and repeated message that the time for change within maternity services is long overdue (DOH, 1993).

Maternity services should reflect the real needs of families.

The goal should no longer be solely prevention of perinatal death, but recognition of the need for confidence and competence in parenting. Only then will women emerge from childbearing with a sense of emotional and physical well-being.

References

Balaskas J, Gordon Y (1990) *Waterbirth*. London: Unwin.

Boxall JF, Whitby C (1989) Who is holding the baby? *Midwives Chronicle and Nursing Notes*; **12** [1213]: 34–36.

Callanan T (1986) Underwater birth. *Mothering*; **Summer**: 59–61.

Church LK (1989) Waterbirth: one birthing centre's observations. *Journal Nurse Midwifery*; **34**: 165–170.

Corbishley H (1989) Waterbirth Workshop New Generation Information Pack No. 12 Bristol: *Midwives Information Resource Pack* (MIDIRS).

Dear PRF, Mclain BL (1987) Establishment of an intermediate care ward for babies and mothers. *Archives of Disease in Childhood*; **63**: 597–600.

De Costa C, Bullivant V, Pisano K et al. (1992) Midwives clinic. *MIDIRS Midwifery Digest* Jun **2** [2]: 140–141.

DOH (1989) *Caring for People. Community Care in the Next Century and Beyond*. London: HMSO.

DOH (1993) *Changing Childbirth*. Part 1. Report Of The Expert Maternity Group Department Of Health. London: HMSO.

Footner K (1992) Bristol's new birth pool. *MIDIRS Midwifery Digest*. September 1992; **2** [3]: 271–274.

Garland D (1993) Aqua births in Maidstone. *MIDIRS Midwifery Digest*. Mar.; **3** [1]: 56–57.

Gordon Y (1991) Waterbirth: a personal view. *Journal of Maternity & Health*; **16**: 245–250.

House Of Commons Health Select Commitee (1992) *Maternity Services*. Health Committee Second Report. Session 1991–2. London: HMSO.

Jepson C (1989) Water. It can help childbirth. *Nursing Times*; **85** [47]: 74–75.

Klaus MH, Kennell JH (1982) *Parent–Infant Bonding*. St. Louis: CV Mosby.

Lenstrup C, Schantz A, Berget A, Feder E, Rosend H, Hertel J (1987) Warm tub bath during delivery. *Acta Obstetricia et Gynecologia*. Scandinavia; **66** [8]: 709–12.

Liu DTY, Jevons B, Thwaites P (1992) Antenatal care towards the year 2000. *Midwives Chronicle & Nursing Notes*. December 1992: 388–390.

Marlow N (1989) The Use of Water in Labour. Conference Report, Pack 12.

Maternity Services Advisory Committee (1984) *Maternity Care In Action*. Part II Care During Childbirth. London: HMSO.

Milner I (1988) Water baths for pain relief in labour. *Nursing Times*; **84** [1]: 38–40.

Ministry Of Health (1929) *Memorandum on Antenatal Clinics: Their Conduct and Scope*. London: HMSO.

Odent M (1983) Birth under water. *Lancet*; **2** [8365–66]: 1476–7.

Page A (1988) Waterbirth: a study. *Homebirth In Australia*; **19**: 3–5.

Prendeville W, Elbourne D (1989) The third stage of labour: In: Chalmers I, Enkin MW, Keirse MJNC (eds), *A Guide to Effective Care in Pregnancy and Childbirth*, Ch. 56. Oxford: Oxford University Press.

Robinson S (1989) The role of the midwife: opportunities and constraints. In: Chalmers I, Enkin MW, Keirse MJNC (eds), *A Guide To Effective Care In Pregnancy And Childbirth*. Oxford: Oxford University Press, pp 162–180.

Rowntree D (1991) *The Managers Book Of Checklists*. London: Corgi, T Ranswards Publishers.

Royal College Of Obstetricians & Gynaecologists (1993) Response To The Report Of Expert Maternity Group: *Changing Childbirth.* 27th Oct 1993. London: Royal College Of Obstetricians & Gynaecologists.

Simkin P (1989) Non-pharmacological methods of pain relief during labour. In: Chalmers I, Enkin MW, Keirse MJNC (eds), *A Guide To Effective Care In Pregnancy And Childbirth,* Ch. 56. Oxford: Oxford University Press.

Siney C (1994) Team effort helps pregnant drug users. *MIDIRS Midwifery Digest.* Jun; **4** [2]: 229–231.

Slome C, Wetherbee H, Daly M, Christenson K, Meglen M, Thiede H (1976) Effectiveness of certified nurse-midwives. A prospective evaluation study. *American Journal Of Obstetrics & Gynaecology;* **124**: 177–182.

Spiby H (1993) Giving complementary therapy with midwifery care for the 1990s. *Midwives Chronicle & Nursing Notes;* February 1993: 38–40.

UKCC (1992a) *Code of Conduct.* United Kingdom Central Council For Nursing, Midwifery & Health Visiting; June 1992.

UKCC (1992b) *Scope Of Professional Practice.* United Kingdom Central Council For Nursing, Midwifery & Health Visiting; June 1992.

13 A taste of your own medicine

Christina Hutcheson Dean

Empowerment, patient satisfaction, therapeutic partnership and self care: These words reflect the mood of nursing in the 1990s. Yet the practice of self-medication, which so clearly expresses their meanings, appears to be the exception and not the rule.

This chapter sets out to explore the values and beliefs which lie behind the practice of self-medication. It describes some of the reasons why the practice is not widespread despite a wealth of researched evidence showing the benefits to patients and staff (Bird, 1990; Simpson and May, 1992; Wood et al., 1992). Within the chapter, a method and guide is given for the implementation of a self-medication programme: this is versatile and can be used in a variety of care settings. The programme is based upon 4 years of successful implementation in a general medical ward of a district general hospital. The ward provides care for 30 patients, most of whom have nursing problems related to acute and chronic illness. There is a high proportion of patients with respiratory disorders, rheumatoid disease or terminal illness.

The nursing staff are a highly committed, enthusiastic and cohesive group who thrive on innovation and change.

Change has occurred as a result of reflection on practice, and the wish to resolve an acknowledged problem. The ward team observed that many patients had poor knowledge and understanding of their drugs; and that little attention was being paid to their education in this aspect of care.

Consider the following scenes:

Scene One

Patient   I've brought all my tablets, nurse, quite a carrier bag full.

Nurse   Goodness, what a lot of drugs, how do you know what to take?

Patient   Well, if my feet are swollen, I take two of these, and there are some I take for pain. I'm supposed to take these three times a day, but I sometimes forget. I just do the best I can.

Scene Two

Nurse   Here are your take home drugs. You take one of these every day, two of these if you have pain, two of these three times a day and this spray if you need it. Do you understand?

Patient   Oh yes, I've got all that. Here's my wife, come to take me home. Thanks for everything.

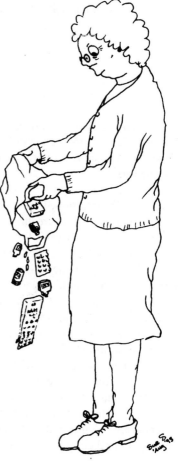

These are scenes familiar to all practising nurses. Familiar, but unacceptable. Unacceptable, because they suggest that the nurse may not be fulfilling her role in the education of patients in their drug regimes. Virginia Henderson's (1978) well loved definition of the role of the nurse states that:

> The unique function of the nurse is to assist the individual, sick or well, in the performance of those activities contributing to health or its recovery, or to peaceful death, that he would perform unaided if he* had the necessary strength, will or knowledge. And to do this in such a way as to help him to gain independence as rapidly as possible.

This definition requires the nurse to help patients in all aspects of daily living. A most elemental aspect of the patient's progress from illness to health and its maintenance lies in his ability to take his medication safely and regularly. This is a reflection of the nurse's belief in the therapeutic partnership that promotes self-care and responsibility.

A therapeutic partnership is a relationship in which patient and nurse work

---

* The use of 'he' for patient, and 'she' for nurse is used for the convenience of illustration, and not to pass covert comment upon power or sexual politics in health care delivery.

together towards cure or the promotion of health. It has been described as 'companionship' on a journey (Campbell, 1984), a 'sharing' of knowledge and skills (Wright, 1990). This gives the patient the ability to make informed choices about health care. When applied to drug administration there can be little choice for the patient who blindly swallows whatever is given to him in hospital or who chooses, without the necessary knowledge, to disregard his drugs once home.

It is the nurse whose unique relationship with the patient best places her to undertake the assessment and education required. As with all care, successful outcomes are based on accurate assessment and planning (Kratz, 1979). Only then can we ensure that the patient is discharged equipped with the knowledge and ability to continue to comply with care.

The philosophy of our ward states, as one of its aims:

> the provision of personalized nursing care to patients and families which promotes self care and responsibility, through partnership.

Self-medication is seen by the team as one of the ways in which this can be achieved. Our aim, through the self-medication programme, is to ensure that each patient is able to

> take his medicine safely and competently, or to make an informed choice not to do so.

This is the key principle underpinning the philosophy of the self-medicating programme. This is supported by Johns (1990), Farrow (1992) and Owen et al. (1987) all of whom describe similar aims for such programmes.

Medication – some facts

- £3 billion of the NHS expenditure was for the provision of drugs in 1991–1992 (Prescription Pricing Authority). Amongst pharmacists a compliance rate of around 80% is considered acceptable to ensure the desired therapeutic effect. However, non-compliance rates of up to 50% have been reported by Evans and Spelman (1983). These two facts together suggest a complex problem and a vast waste of resource.
- Ten per cent of hospital admissions in elderly people are due to drug related incidents such as digoxin overdose (Bliss, 1981).
- Lack of knowledge and understanding contributing to non-compliance increases with age. Hopkins (1990) in his study of a group of patients with rheumatoid disease found that 35% of the patients over the age of 75 expressed no knowledge about their drugs.
- Non-compliance cannot always be related to the patient. It can in part be due to poor education by medical, nursing and pharmacy staff. For example, Taylor and Tunstell (1991) found little difference between professionals and patients in both knowledge of, and technique in using, metered dose inhalers.
- Bird (1990) found that compliance and patient satisfaction are increased when a programme of self-medication has been implemented.

- Meadows (1990) showed that patients transferring from mental health institutions to rehabilitation homes are able, after a programme, to take their medications safely and competently.
- In a small study of patients in the author's setting (1992), over 80% of patients expressed improved satisfaction and understanding of their drug regime.

A study of the above and of the other widely available research will lead nurses to the conclusion that the benefits of self-medication far outweigh any disadvantages. The purpose of this chapter is to promote a positive approach and to examine the practicalities. A consideration of the factors involved in non-compliance, however, should be given as they have a relevance to practice.

Factors involved in non-compliance

1 Patients' lack of understanding of condition.
2 Lack of understanding of drugs.
3 Complexity of regime.
4 Physiological factors.
5 Unintentional non-compliance.
6 Current practice in hospital.
7 Shorter hospital stays.

Patients' lack of understanding of condition

It may be surprising that a considerable number of patients do not know the condition for which their drugs are being taken. They may well be able to describe their symptoms but do not know what causes them (Bird, 1990). If the purpose of a drug regime is not known the motivation for compliance may be diminished.

Lack of understanding of drugs

Information given about drugs in a traditional setting is often restricted to answering the odd question in the course of a drugs round. This is assuming the patient dares to interrupt the busy nurse. If patients are to succeed in complying with regimes they need to know the actions of their drugs, duration of courses and timings. They also need to know the side effects which may occur and the action to take if they do. This does not lead to a vast increase in visits to medical staff but rather to rational action by the patient.

Complexity of regime

There is a need to simplify drug regimes if compliance is to be improved. This may necessitate the omission of some drugs in order to ensure that the most important medications are taken. Compliance is decreased if more than four different drugs are required, or if each drug needs to be taken more than once or twice daily.

However, if a once-daily drug is forgotten, then therapy is being omitted for a 24-h period (Parkin et al., 1976).

Physiological factors

Factors such as poor eyesight, forgetfulness, confusion and restricted mobility can contribute to non-compliance.

These factors are compounded if there is complexity in regimes, inadequate education and poorly labelled or non-accessible containers. In the elderly there may also be altered sensitivity to drugs and a high incidence of reaction (Cope, 1988).

Unintentional non-compliance

This may occur when an individual forgets to take a tablet (which of us doesn't?) or be unaware of the need to renew a prescription.

Current practice in hospital

The role of the nurse in the storage and administration of drugs means there is little attention paid to the education of patients. There is usually minimal time available for education during a traditional 'drug round' and the nurse's attention is focused on the safe administration of the drugs. Rarely is time set aside, as a planned intervention, for educating patients about their drugs. Drug rounds also poorly reflect the normal pattern of drug taking once the patient is home. Individuals usually prefer to link their drug regime to either their meal times or work patterns.

The education patients receive about drugs prior to discharge is usually limited to the last 10 minutes of their stay. In the excitement and relief at going home it is unlikely that much of the information is either understood or processed for future use (Wood et al., 1992). The patient is often only given instructions and no attempt is made to test recall and understanding. It is hardly surprising the patient arrives home and finds himself unable to comply.

Current practice in educating patients in relation to drugs does not emphasize the need to prepare the patient for home which other components of care attract. For example, the patient who has had a stroke demands a multidisciplinary approach to ensure his safe transfer from hospital to home. This involves medical and nursing input and the involvement of other therapies, notably physiotherapy and occupational therapy. Many weeks of care may be needed to enable the patient to cope at home but medication will generally receive minimal attention. This may be satisfactory if carers are available, but what if the patient lives alone? The ability to comply with drugs may be the deciding factor in the maintenance of the patient's future health.

Shorter hospital stays

The trend towards shorter hospital stays may have a greater impact than imagined on patient non-compliance. The time for a patient to learn about his drugs may be limited to only a few days.

It is clear from a discussion of the above factors, that a programme of self-administration would be helpful to the majority of patients. As well as the benefits of increased knowledge and compliance there are less obvious but valuable advantages. Patients able to self-medicate in hospital are able to retain a sense of control. This is important for every one of us. Panic and anxiety soon set in if we feel we have lost control of our own destiny. Historically, the patient has given up control when he takes on the patient role and devolves his responsibility to the professionals (Parsons, 1951). This does still occur but is becoming less of the 'norm' as individuals become empowered. Where a self-care model for nursing is in use then the education necessary to give control becomes an integral part of that care.

Care models such as Orem (1980) and Roper et al. (1980) imply a transition from dependence to independence with nursing interventions designed to assist. Medication is no exception.

A therapeutic nurse/patient partnership is based on co-operation (Peplau, 1952). This is evident and emphasized where self-medication programmes exist. The patient uses the knowledge and expertise of the nurse to help him to maintain motivation and to speed recovery. Patients able to self-medicate are confident in their ability to continue to comply at home. As with most aspects of care, improved information giving, tailored to the individual's needs, leads to improved satisfaction with care (Bird, 1990).

Implementation – a guide for a successful self-medication programme

The successful implementation of a self-medication programme is based on the user's perception and belief in the value of that system. If this is achieved, the organizational detail will fall into place. It is helpful if the programme is seen as an integral part of the chosen system of care delivery.

The concepts of therapeutic partnerships and empowerment imply control and informed choices for patients. For nurses to retain control over the administration of all patients' drugs is in many ways contrary to these beliefs.

Successful change is based upon planning and preparation. A period of 6–12 months may be needed to prepare everyone involved for fundamental change (Wright, 1990). Change strategies abound, but rarely do people fit into them!

Time is needed for staff to read and study the proposals and the available researched evidence. The objectives of patient competence, compliance and satisfaction may need clarification and discussion before being accepted by all. Time given to study, discussion of roles, worries and fears will facilitate a positive team approach and ensure a smooth transition to new practice. Enthusiasm, tenacity and broad shoulders are required by the change agent.

In practical terms, it is entirely reasonable that the actual implementation of the programme should follow a systematic approach known and used by nurses, that is, the nursing process of:

> **assessment;**
> **planning;**
> **implementation;**
> **evaluation.**

Assessment

Assessment should be undertaken by the nurse and the ward pharmacist, and include the following factors:

- Understanding of illness.
- Knowledge of current drugs.
- What drugs are for.
- What actions they have.
- Side effects.
- Motivation.
- Ability to read and interpret instructions.
- Ability to manage packaging.
- Physical factors.

This assessment can be carried out during the taking of a nursing history. In conjunction with the pharmacist's assessment, the patient's consent to take part in the programme is sought. The patient's consent is also an indication of his motivation. With his agreement the patient is assigned to one of the following four stages of the programme which span the continuum:

unable to self-medicate $\longleftrightarrow$ able to self-medicate

Stage one	Unable to self-medicate, because of poor knowledge, confusion, or present ill state.
Stage two	Able to self-medicate with help and supervision. Can open bottles, read and follow instructions. Can state drug action but needs further education.
Stage three	Able to self-medicate with minimal supervision. Complies with stage two. Able to state drug actions, duration and timing and side effects. Requires only check before taking drugs. Can record accurately.
Stage four	Able to self-medicate independently.

Planning

The assessment data are used to plan the appropriate goals and interventions which will result in the patient moving ultimately to stage four. These goals are clearly identified on the patient's care plan which is kept at the bedside.

Time is allocated on the care plan for teaching and assessing the patient on a daily basis. This time should be separate from the drug round as this enhances the one-to-one relationship, and means that the actual drug round does not become overlong. The pharmacist visits the ward each day and also assesses the patient's progress. As the prescription sheet is kept by the patient's bedside, medical staff become involved in the education of patients, giving explanations of changes as and when they occur. The medical staff have been enthusiastic in their support of the programme. Written information and any necessary charts which the patient needs can also be given at this planned time.

Implementation

The drugs are kept in a central locking trolley with separate drawers labelled for each patient. There are other ways of storing drugs (described later) and no one way is superior to another. Drugs are dispensed from the pharmacy with 7 days' supply in individually labelled containers showing the patient's name, drug name and dose, and instructions. When the patient goes home, the drugs are topped up to give a further 7 days' supply. A considerable amount of pharmacy time is required to do this and negotiation with pharmacy is required at the outset. Although the drugs are kept in a locked trolley, patients self-medicating at stage four have access to their drugs simply by request. Drug rounds for other patients are carried out at mealtimes so this usually coincides with the patient's wishes.

In practice, patients at stage one have their drugs administered in the traditional manner with additional information being given. Encouragement is also given to ask questions. Patients at stage two are given total supervision at each drug administration. The time used for education and teaching away from the drug round is assessed for its success by questioning and discussion at the time of drug administration. When the patient can demonstrate proficiency both verbally and in practice in taking his medicines he progresses to stage three. At this stage he requires only minimal supervision. Perhaps he may be asked not to take his drugs until a final check is made by his nurse. When the nurse and patient are satisfied that all the criteria set at assessment have been met, the patient will then be able to self-medicate independently.

Record keeping

This should be kept as simple as possible. In the author's experience, after several trials, a record which is used by patients, medical and nursing staff alike is ideal. This lessens chances of duplication and problems with transcribing. A prescription sheet which is a different colour from that used by the rest of the hospital makes it readily identifiable in the pharmacy. A copy of a suitable prescription sheet is given below.

Space is available for 12 regular items to allow for changes during the patient's stay. Times are breakfast, lunch, tea and bedtime to accommodate a more normal lifestyle. There is space for 'as necessary drugs' and 'once only' drugs. Whoever gives the drugs, be it patient or nurse, signs the appropriate column.

MID CHESHIRE HOSPITALS – **LEIGHTON HOSPITAL, WARD TWO**
MEDICATION RECORD FOR:

| PATIENT'S NAME, ADDRESS, DATE OF BIRTH AND REGISTRATION NUMBER – OR AFFIX ADDRESSOGRAPH. | ALLERGIES AND DRUG SENSITIVITIES |
| | DATE OF ADMISSION |

MEDICATION WILL BE PRESCRIBED BY THE DOCTOR AND ADMINISTERED BY
NURSING STAFF/PATIENT (Delete as appropriate)

| CONSULTANT | DOCTOR | | PRIMARY NURSE | | PHARMACIST | |

REGULAR MEDICATION		Day and → Date							
DRUG	Route	B'fast							
DOSE AND INSTRUCTIONS		Lunch							
		Tea							
DOCTORS SIGNATURE	Pharm.								
		Bed							
DRUG	Route	B'fast							
DOSE AND INSTRUCTIONS		Lunch							
		Tea							
DOCTORS SIGNATURE	Pharm.								
		Bed							

Evaluation

The success of a programme is monitored by evaluation. Questionnaires have been used to elicit patient satisfaction with the system. Over 80% are positive. Patients being prepared for home are no longer given their drugs with verbal and written instructions only but are asked to tell their nurse what they are to take, how often and why. Although our current practice does not follow up patients at home, it is envisaged that a pilot scheme to do this will be in place in the near future.

It is not always necessary for every patient to be able to self-medicate independently. One of the insights gained from the programme has been to identify patients who will need help to comply once home. The necessary support can then be put into place prior to discharge. For example:

Fred has a chronic chest disorder and diabetes mellitus. After frequent admissions it was decided to help him to self-medicate in case non-compliance was contributing to his frequent admissions. It was found that he was unable to read at all. As he attends a day centre, provision for a 7-day dispenser was made. This is filled weekly by his local chemist and delivered to the day centre where the staff administer his drugs to him.

Patients with difficulties in opening bottles can be identified and issued with suitable containers such as those with butterfly tops, or those with non-childproof tops. Families can receive the necessary help and instruction if they are identified as the main carers involved.

The programme has raised awareness of the need to give patients more knowledge and help with drugs. Whilst compliance and safety are paramount, there is an immense satisfaction in seeing the patient who is confident in his knowledge, understanding and ability to self-medicate. He in turn feels in control and able to make a contribution to his recovery and sustained improvement. Wood et al. (1992) found, at the follow-up of patients who had taken part in a self-medication programme in hospital, only 6% had made errors compared with 47% in the control group.

Follow-up is a subject requiring further study. In my own area, nurses telephone their patients routinely 3–5 days after discharge to monitor their general progress. Queries about drugs do still continue to be made and are usually easily resolved.

Roles and attitudes

A multidisciplinary approach to self-medication is essential for its successful implementation. This approach must involve the patient as a partner in his care rather than a recipient of that care (Kendrick, 1991). Otherwise all the time and effort invested may result in a perfectly compliant patient in hospital who returns home and chooses not to comply! Medication is not always seen as part of holistic care but rather as a separate entity. Effective discharge policies demand planning for home from day 1 of admission but preparation for drug taking usually occurs in the last 10 minutes of the patient's stay.

The patient

Historically, the patient has been seen as someone who takes on a passive role having once crossed the threshold of the ward door (Pearson and Vaughan, 1986). The expectation has been that his clothes, often his identity and certainly his drugs are removed from him on admission and he allows himself to be 'cared for' by the knowledgeable professional. There are many reasons why this is so. Being ill gives a person an exemption from his usual role but in order to maintain this new role he has to give up independence and accept care from others (Parsons, 1951). This can mean that individuals who are perfectly capable of self-medicating and may have been successfully doing so prior to admission, lose their feelings of control. This is both unnecessary and non-therapeutic. Many patients are still unaware of their rights and responsibilities, but this is beginning to change.

The patient's role in successful self-medication programmes is crucial and needs to be seen in relation to personalized and individual care. The patient needs to perceive himself as the principal player with the professionals as the supporting cast.

There is evidence to suggest that some patients do not wish to be self reliant whilst in hospital and prefer to have their medication given by nursing staff (Thomas, 1992). They do not wish to be bothered whilst in hospital, or are fearful of making mistakes. 'Nurse knows best' is often quoted as a reason for not self-medicating. If these patients feel unable to administer their drugs whilst in hospital with support, there seems little likelihood of success once home.

Medical staff

Many medical staff are enthusiastic in their support for programmes which help patients to comply with drug regimes. Self-medication encourages discussion with patients. Where such programmes are in place it is almost impossible for medical staff to change or review drugs without interaction taking place with the patient.

Some medical staff take the view that the patient does not need to be involved in his medication other than to be sure to take it. This may indicate an unwillingness to participate in the extra discussion and explanations required. As such, this view is shortsighted as benefits may include the non-readmission of the patient. It is easier to say 'take this three times a day and you will feel better tomorrow/in a week/soon'. This attitude reflects the view that knowledge is power. After all, would you take a tablet without knowing its likely action or side effects? Of course not.

Medical staff are important in a self-medication programme. Their initial contact in prescribing medication sets the scene for the other staff involved in its implementation.

Pharmacist

Almost universally, pharmacists take the view that self-medication programmes are an excellent means to promoting compliance (Cope, 1988). The pharmacist's role lies in education, along with nurses and medical staff, of the patient and his family through a variety of teaching tools such as charts, calendars or 7-day dispensers. It is useful for the pharmacist to be involved in the initial assessment or selection of suitable patients. The pharmacist has access to, and knowledge of many of the 'tricks of the trade' which help ensure understanding and compliance.

Our pharmacist sees patients on the ward every day, thus encouraging questioning and communication. Patients on a self-medication programme have time spent explaining their drug actions, side effects, timing and record keeping. Charts can be supplied if needed. All patients are seen every day, whether on the programme or not. Some patients ask to join in based on hearing other patients talk to the pharmacist.

The pharmacist has a role, as a member of the ward team, in communicating with nursing and medical staff giving help in the rationalization of regimes. Most patients can cope with an optimum of four drugs at any one time, preferably on a once only or twice daily basis. This may mean omitting some drugs in favour of ensuring compliance with those essential to the patient's recovery, and the maintenance of health once home. The involvement of the pharmacist in the programme has meant an increase in pharmacist/patient contact which is most welcome (Corrigan, 1989).

Nurse

The nurse has a unique role in administering drugs, as the named person responsible for the care and custody of drugs. To relinquish this responsibility to patients can be a cause for concern for some nurses. The UKCC issued standards (UKCC, 1992) for the care and administration of drugs which, if followed, ensure the nurse's accountability is not compromised.

The nurse has a relationship with the patient based on mutual trust. The implementation of personalized care systems allows the development of a therapeutic partnership within which she can assess, plan, implement and evaluate that care with the patient. She is in a position to enable the patient to understand a drug regime, to help him to learn to take and record his own medication, and to reinforce the motivation for doing so. In so doing she also increases her own knowledge and understanding of drugs.

As a teacher, the nurse can use her knowledge, imagination, enthusiasm and the sound principles of learning (Gerrish, 1990). Her role extends to the family and to the carers if they are to be the ones responsible for medication once the patient is home. The nurse is the facilitator who enables the patient to make informed choices. Her attitude will influence the patient probably more than other professionals because of her prolonged and close contact with him.

Nurses are not renowned for their success in forward planning (Gillis, 1988). As a workforce, the pressure is often upon them to get today's work done. Yet time invested at an early part of the patient's stay may be time saved later when the patient is able to control and self-administer drugs safely and without supervision.

Other considerations

Controlled drugs

There seems little reason why a patient proficient in administering his drugs should be denied the right to self-administer controlled drugs. After all, he would do so in his own home situation. There are additional constraints in hospital because of the legal requirements for storage and administration of controlled drugs. This should not, in itself, preclude any patient from taking part in a self-medication programme. The patient should feel that he can ask for his controlled drugs to be administered at the appropriate times for him and his nurse should make them available to him (Cottrell, 1990).

Case study

Joan, aged 59, had many admissions during the course of her illness. Sadly she had cancer of the lung. Throughout the early part of her illness she delighted in being able to self-medicate, including taking her own controlled drugs. She said she felt this maintained her independence, and helped her to be in control. When she grew weaker she herself asked the nursing staff to take over for her. This is surely an example of partnership and demonstrates autonomous choice for the patient.

Risks

Drug administration involves risk, as does any other component of care. The management of risk requires the identification of potential problems and their removal or reduction. Accurate assessment of individual patients should minimize the risk of over or under dosage. Some categories of patients, such as those with confusion, dementia, or some psychiatric problems, may need to be excluded from programmes. If, however, mistakes are going to occur, it is better that it should be in hospital where help is at hand than at home. Constant supervision and assistance should be provided until the patient demonstrates an ability to self-medicate competently.

Storage of drugs

Some centres operate a no lock system (Bird, 1988), as the drugs are then in the control of the patient without his having to ask. In these circumstances it is wise to look at the client group that the ward or unit serves, to minimize the risk of abuse. In any event, patients are asked to keep their drugs out of sight either in lockers or in handbags.

It is possible to use locking containers for which the patient holds the key and which can be attached to the required locker by means of a simple wing nut and bolt system. This allows the use of the containers wherever they are needed in the ward.

If a central locking system is used, the drug trolley should be compartmentalized with named sections for each patient, and it should be known that the patients may ask for their drug container whenever they wish, and do not need to wait for drug rounds.

Patient controlled analgesia

This is in use in many surgical areas and can be seen as a form of self-medication. Analgesia, usually in the form of narcotic drugs, is given by syringe driver which the patient operates by means of a push button. A measured dose is delivered and a lock-out system prevents over dosage during a predetermined time period. Evaluations from patients for this type of patient controlled analgesia indicate a high level of satisfaction, with patients preferring this to having to wait for injections. They feel in control, neither having to wait for, nor to ask for analgesia. A survey in 1993 on the surgical unit at Leighton Hospital indicated 82% of patients preferred this system (Edwards, 1993).

Dallison (1991) studied the use of patient controlled oral analgesia following patient controlled intravenous analgesia. Patients were given a supply of 30 Coproxamol tablets to be used over 4 days. Patients used less analgesia, and it was noted that the tablets were taken at times which suited the patients, and rarely at the conventional drug round times.

Residential or nursing home care

If individuals are to continue to maintain their independent status as far as possible when in residential or nursing home care there seems no reason why they should not self-medicate. Guidelines should be available to promote this and should incorporate the principles of assessment, planning, implementation and evaluation (Cheshire County Council, 1992).

Liability

Traditional methods of administering medicines in hospital are aimed at keeping the patient and the nurse safe. Adequate planning and co-operation is essential, and a local policy for self-medication should be agreed with medical, nursing and pharmacy staff. Written policies and procedures should be made available and provided these are adhered to and patients are accurately assessed and supervised then problems should not arise.

Conclusion

Self-medication programmes are rather like the production of a play. The characters are the patients, nurses, doctors, pharmacists and families. All have roles to play. Like most productions, planning and practice are vital if the performance is to be an acclaimed success.

All nurses have a responsibility to help their patients to safely take their medication by themselves or with the help of others. For many patients, medication represents a major component of their care. The nurse who sees medication as an integral part of holistic care and who invests time to assess and implement a programme for her patient will be well rewarded. There is satisfaction for the patient who is able to comply and for the nurse who has contributed to such positive outcomes.

As the notion of empowerment grows, self-medication programmes will assume even greater importance. Perhaps then self-medication will become the rule rather than the exception. There is a wealth of research evidence available to us, of which only a small fraction has been cited here. Nurses owe it to their patients to act upon it.

Scene three

Patient   'I'm going home today, nurse, shall I go through my drugs with you and tell you what I have to take, when and why? Then you'll be sure I know what I'm doing when I get home.'

Nurse   'Well done. I'll phone you in 2 or 3 days time to check that all's well.'

References

Bird C (1988) Taking their own medicine. *Nursing Times*; **84** [45]: 28–32.
Bird C (1990) A prescription for self help. *Nursing Times*; **86** [43]: 52–55.
Bliss MR (1981) Prescribing for the elderly. *British Medical Journal*; **283**: 203–206.
Campbell, AV (1984) *Moderated Love*. London: SPCK.
Cheshire County Council (1992) *Guidelines for Self Medication in Residential Homes*.
Cope A (1988) The role of the hospital pharmacist in the care of the elderly. *Pharmaceutical Journal Hospital Pharmaceutical Suppl. HS*; **March 12**: 16–18.
Corrigan MS (1989) Primary pharmacy – a patient's self help service. *The Pharmaceutical Journal*; 7 October: 458–460.
Cottrell N (1990) The view from the pharmacy. *Nursing Times*; **86** [43]: 55–57.
Dallison A (1991) Self-administration of oral pain relief. *Nursing*; **4** [35]: 30–31.
Edwards C, Chriscoli B (1993) *Patients' Views on Patient Controlled Analgesia*. Leighton Hospital, Crewe.
Evans L, Spelman M (1983). The problem of non-compliance with drug therapy. *Drugs*; **26** [1]: 63–76.
Farrow S (1992) How much do they know? *Professional Nurse*; **November**: 118–124.
Gerrish CA (1990) Purposes, values and objectives in adult education – the post-basic perspective. *Nurse Education Today*. April; **10** [2]: 118–124.
Gillis I (1988) *Human Behaviour in Illness*. London: Faber and Faber.
Henderson V (1978) The concept of nursing. *Journal of Advanced Nursing*; **3**: 113–130.
Hopkins R (1990) Sans awareness. *Nursing Times*; **86** [30]: 50–51.
Johns C (1990) Steps to self medication. *Nursing Times*; **86** [11]: 40–41.
Kendrick K (1991) Partners in passing: ethical aspects of nursing the dying patient. *Journal of Advances in Health and Nursing Care*; **1** [1]: 11–26.
Kratz C (1979) *The Nursing Process*. London: Ballière Tindall.
Meadows C (1990) Keep taking the tablets. *Nursing Times*; **86** [24]: 69–70.
Orem D (1980) *Nursing Concepts of Practice*. New York: McGraw Hill.
Owen DS, James DW, Howard P (1987) Self medication scheme on a rheumatology ward. *British Journal of Pharmaceutical Practice*; October: 386–390.
Parkin DM, Henney CR, Quirk J, Crooks J (1976) Deviation from prescribed drug treatment after discharge. *British Medical Journal*; **2**: 686–688.
Parsons T (1951) *The Social System*. New York: Free Press.
Pearson A, Vaughan B (1986) *Nursing Models for Practice*. London: Heinemann.
Peplau H (1952) *Interpersonal Relations in Nursing*. New York: Putmans Sons.
Prescription Pricing Authority. (1991–1992) *Annual Report*.
Roper N, Logan WN, Tierney AJ (1980) *The Elements of Nursing*. Edinburgh: Churchill Livingstone.
Simpson J, May LG (1992) Self administration in hospital – towards better compliance. *Hospital Pharmacy Practice*. January, 30–33.
Taylor D, Tunstell P (1991) Metered dose inhalers – a system for assessing technique in patients and health professionals. *Pharmaceutical Journal*; 18 May: 626–627.
Thomas E (1992) Self medication. *Nursing*; **5** [2]: 26–27.
UKCC (1992) *Standards for the Administration of Drugs*. October.
Wood SJ, Calvert RT, Acomb C, Kay EA (1992) A self medication scheme for elderly patients improves compliance with medication regimes. *International Journal of Pharmacy Practice*; August: 240–241.
Wright SG (1990) *My Patient – My Nurse*. Harrow: Scutari Press.

Index